The Essentials of
IRIDOLOGY
The Eyes: Windows to Health

LaDean Griffin

Cover Photo by Kirsten Tenney
http://adeliaphotography.weebly.com/

TABLE OF CONTENTS

INTRODUCTION

Iridology is not a new discovery, but rather dates back to the twelfth century. Shepherds down through the ages have examined the eyes of their sheep to check health and to cull out the weak ones. Stockmen still examine cattle eyes to determine the general health of their livestock, by observing whether the eyes are bright and vibrant or dull and lifeless.

The formal medical study of the eye probably began with Hippocrates, as did so much of the study of human anatomy. Most authors agree that the study of the iris of the eye began with Ignatz Von Peczely in 1866. As a boy in Bulgaria, he noticed that a pet owl with a broken leg also had a mark on the iris of the eye corresponding to the break. As the leg healed, this spot grew smaller. This interested Von Peczely, who later became a medical doctor. As a doctor in Bulgaria he studied people being admitted to the hospital, drawing pictures of their irises. Upon their release from the hospital, he again drew pictures, and then compared the two pictures. This prompted him to write a book on his studies entitled *Discoveries in the Realm of Nature and the Art of Healing.* Dr. Von Peczely also made the first iridology chart and discovered that the parts of the iris corresponded with parts of the body and the organs. He outlined this relationship on his iridology chart.

Dr. Von Peczely's work inspired other European doctors like Dr. Nils Lilinquist of Sweden, who first noticed the effects of drugs on the iris of the eye. Other European iridologists were inspired to further the work and bring it to the New World. It has been slow to start in the United States, but because of the work of people like Dr. Bernard Jensen and myself, the work continues to grow. Books like Dr. Jensen's *The Science and Practice of Iridology* volumes 1 and 2, and my book *Eyes the Windows of the Body and the Soul*, as well as extensive lecturing across the country by myself and others, has acquainted many people with iridology. Although in 1978 there were probably only a few hundred iridologists in the United States, at present there are thousands of lay iridologists. Everyone who hears the principles of iridology related to corrective diet, herbs, and vitamins and applies them in his own life eventually proves such principles to himself. The interest by the medical community over the 10 years that I have been lecturing has been astounding. Over the past four years it was rare when I did not have medical doctors, chiropractors, nurses, and pharmacists in my classes, and their particular interest seem to be in iridology.

My contribution to the work already done in the history of iridology has been to show how to relate iridology to the use of herbs and a mild food diet. Improvement can be recognized simply by the way a person feels as he learns herbs and a corrective diet. With the use of iridology he can also watch the changes as they take place in his eyes. This is a Marvel and a wonder to behold, for as the body heals the eyes change like a kaleidoscope. When such results can be achieved, the logic of a mild food diet and the use of herbs is sound and iridology proves the truth of both.

The use of drugs by established medical methods for healing has too long proven ineffective. It was previously assumed that drugs were all that was needed, and in the beginning the whole idea of finding a wonder drug to solve the world's physical problems met with little resistance. Everyone liked the idea, "Break all the rules of health and diet; don't worry, the doctor will give you a little pill, or when needed cut you open, and he will take all the responsibility for your health." However, thinking people everywhere have become disenchanted with this concept, as well as with the drugs themselves. They have come to the conclusion that drugs are alien to the natural physiology of man concerning the human body and that all the rules of physical laws have been broken in a search for alternative solutions. Meanwhile, a new, yet old, science has risen to popularity and returned to the herb kingdom for the answers. However, those who are thinking even more deeply are recognizing that the real answer does not lie in medicine of any kind but rather in obedience to the laws of nature. Only then will man be free of the pain of disease. Preventative medicine has become the real solution.

In order for iridology to be of value to the layperson so that he may be able to analyze the inside of his body, it is essential to understand how to use iridology specifically in conjunction with herbs and correct diet.

When my study of iridology began almost 40 years ago, it appeared to be an excellent method of analysis, but it bothered me greatly that no one seemed to know how to make any health changes register on the iris of the eye rapidly. Changes occurred more quickly, however, and were noted when the diet was changed to either a vegetarian or fruitarian diet. Even the combination of vegetarian and fruitarian diets proved significant changes, but it was a slow process of lifestyle change, in some cases. Orthodox medicine was expanding rapidly at the time. Science, through chemical research, was promising new wonder drugs for every disease. This promise was carrying people on the crest of a wave that was later to overshadow most alternative medicines. When a headache could be stopped in minutes with aspirin, and upset stomach could be instantly relieved, and pain could be halted in its ongoing process, it seemed without question that everyone was deeply inspired with the magic of drug therapy.

My childhood background in natural living could not be overcome, however, by the fashion of the day. My strict Mormon background forbid the use of coffee, tea, tobacco, and alcohol, but my home training went even further. I felt guilty if I took an aspirin or ate sugar that was not raw or flour that was not whole wheat.

I always felt somehow that there was a food or plant that could help to overcome any health problem, with the exception of an organic, inherent genetic birth defect. It had always seemed to me that broken laws were the causes of disease. If this is true, certainly a merciful God should have made a medicine to overcome or at least relieve disease. Since all of life is based on the principle of repentance, or trial and error, it seems to me medicine that any person can find and use is more useful in many ways than synthetic or man-made medicine. Over the centuries man has learned which herbs to use for different disease by both study and by inspiration. Orthodox medicine has probed with laser-like accuracy, penetrating the microscopic agent of diseased tissue and even the DNA molecule. With all the technical pinpointing in medicine, the rest of the whole body becomes the blind spot. Herbs, on the other hand, influence the entire body rather than a specific area. Aside from the poisons of the drugs, treating isolated areas of the body seems to be the greatest weakness of Orthodox medicine. By comparison, herbal remedies are always gentler and safer, with no side effects.

One of the main reasons for the great hope of iridology is that as the body begins to deteriorate in any given area, the iris perceives not only the deterioration but the extent to which the disease is involved. With the perspective of the iris a person must always maintain a constant vigil in order to deter deterioration, and at all times an all out program must be performed to overcome the invading disease. The advantage becomes twofold: prevention or correction and restoration of health. The eyes are truly the windows of the body. Every error, injury, or pathological disturbance in the body finds its way to the windows, where we can peer in to discover the uttermost dark, secret and hidden places. As the body heals through correct principle, the eyes will change like a kaleidoscope, a wondrous miracle to behold. Serious health problems appear on the eye long before symptoms begin to cause alarm, and with a disease like cancer, by the time help is sought, it is already too late.

Medical science as a whole has not accepted iridology as a true science because medical drugs do not heal the body; therefore, this beautiful change in the eyes as repairs are made cannot be experienced by Orthodox methods. If medical science were to use nature's methods they would soon learn as I have that the eye is a wonderful x-ray, and that God did not place us on earth so that the only way we could find out what was wrong with our bodies was to be cut open or have all kinds of fluids run through our veins so that our insides could be photographed. No, he put windows on us. It has been evident to many who have learned about iridology that with the use of herbs and mild foods, the eye changes as health is restored. The iris of the eye demonstrates places where bones have been broken, where surgery has been performed, and where glands are functioning and where they are not. You can determine where parasites are present in the body and in what areas they have accumulated. It can even be determined whether a person has taken drugs and where in the body they are lodged. The vitality, strength, and weakness of a body is evidenced in the iris. Anemia or an over toxic condition may also be seen in the iris, along with accumulation of waste such as cancerous tumors, arthritis, etc. When a person is nervous, it can be determined just how nervous by the number of nerve rings on the iris. Inherently weak places in the body, or where the body is most likely to break down, are evident in the iris long before that area finally does break down.

Man has devised an instrument called an oscilloscope. When this electrical instrument is hooked to an automobile or many other electrical or mechanical devices using electricity, electrical images will appear on the screen as electrical impulses. These impulses allow the electrician, engineer, or mechanic, to tell just how the device is working or if it is malfunctioning. It will show any weak or strong impulses. It will also show the rhythm, speed, and timing of each device. Man has also attached sensing devices to the body of an astronaut and sent him thousands of miles into space. Information is radioed back to mission control for doctors to monitor. Doctors can tell his heart rate, blood pressure, body temperature, respiration, and general body condition. It can be determined when he exercises, his strength, and his endurance. Today you can walk into any hospital and see diagnostic equipment attached to patients. In the nursery this research appears to be cruel and brutal, especially when it has to be accompanied by all of the antibiotics and all of the drugs which slow down and even inhibiting the process of healing. If it is possible for man to make such devices is it not more probable that God, in his infinite wisdom could have put a screen on us that made it unnecessary to go through all of the pain of diagnostic tests? The eyes are literally the oscilloscopes of the body and infinitely more. When medical science learns how to heal the body of chronic disease, it will learn that this is true.

In my discussion of iridology, my intention will be, to show you the main things to look for and some of the discoveries I have found that others have not. Some of the weak places showing on the eye may be inherent, some are caused by injury, others we will just call weakness, acquired by either a flaw in personal character, choice, or environment. They all show up in the same way, and since this analytical study has nothing to do with the physique, you will not be able to determine which of the four is the cause in anyone – with the exception of yourself. Personality character weaknesses that cause illness will be discussed in the first chapter.

In my books *Is Any Sick Among You?* and *No Side Effects; The Return to Herbal Medicine,* fasting, the use of mild foods, correct food combinations, home remedies with herbs and vitamins, and care for the colon are discussed. The layperson can learn to be specific in determining what is wrong in the body. To learn iridology, without learning what to do for what is seen, would be of little value to anyone other than to play games, and playing games could hurt more than it could help. As you begin to take your first look into the body, you need a good eye loupe and flashlight, in order to see.

To see one's own eyes, an eye loupe is placed directly against the eye, using a magnifying mirror in front of the loupe while in a bright light. Other concave mirror devices are also on the market to see into one's own eyes. A darker shade than the color of the eye will manifest itself as an outline on the colon, stomach, autonomic wreath and peripheral, or outside line of the iris. Noting the fineness or looseness of the texture of the eyes makes it easy to determine general strength and the ability to heal. Anything, other than darker lines on colon, stomach, autonomic wreath and peripheral line areas, showing in the iris of the eye is disease or inherent weakness. When inherent weakness, there will be a darker shadow than the color of the eye, either in a shadow or a bowed out place which we will call a lesion.

CHAPTER 1

WEAKNESS

Loose Texture

Fine Texture

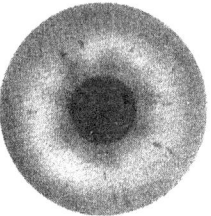

Fine Texture with Black Spots

Inherent weakness can develop into illness. The most dangerous weaknesses to have are the ones that affect the heart, liver, kidneys, and the glands. Many weaknesses are related or interrelated and move along the body like a chain reaction, other weaknesses are unrelated, and there are times when a person can live to a ripe old age with a lot of weaknesses that never connect. The inherent, inborn kind of weakness can sometimes be changed by diet and correct living. The person who is very weak inherently cannot get away with the abuse that a stronger, more healthy person might give his body.

Personality weaknesses may also cause illness. A person who is too sensitive, who has too much self-pity or who is not sensitive enough and doesn't care about others, has a personality weakness. A rebellious, stubborn, or destructive person, or a weak willed person who allows others to do his deciding for him and accepts wrong choices in diet, also fits this category. The indecisive person who can't make up his mind and will usually walk the middle of the road, or a negative person who is pessimistic or a worrying type certainly have weaknesses. Even the individuals who are unable to give or receive love, or even those types who are unable to accept things as they are, need to strengthen those weaknesses. All such types with personality weaknesses are prone to illness. There are those who consider that if they had made the world, they would have done most things differently. They are never able to accept things, the world, or other people as they are. People with inferiority complexes also fit this category.

Then there is the idealist. It is with difficulty that the idealist lives with weakness or imperfection, in himself or his fellow men. To begin with, as he grows up, he believes in himself and everyone else. As he becomes disappointed in others or himself or his weaknesses, he is shattered. When those he loves or respects disappoint him, he can become very ill, sometimes causing a nervous breakdown or even death, such as the woman with very high ideals who had a complete breakdown when she discovered that her husband was sleeping with other women. She was unable to accept him on the basis of this even though she loved him with all her heart, but her standards were not low enough to allow infidelity of any kind, let alone adultery. If she had remained with him, it could have killed her. For good health, it is better for birds of a feather to flock together. Sometimes those of idealistic temperament, who not quite measure up themselves, will place the standard of perfection on another person: a parent, a grandparent, a church leader, a friend, or a business partner. When that person falls, their whole world, testimony, sense of right and wrong, love and forgiveness, suddenly crashes about their feet.

There are those who wish to achieve greatness, but because of a parent's bad example or the circumstances in which they have found themselves, they are never quite sure how much of that parent's traits have been handed down to them. They do not quite ever believe they can make it. They either become resigned to living with mediocrity or they are continually torn. There have been many parents who have had to live out the rest of their lives with broken health or have gone to an early grave because a wayward child has broken their heart and spirit.

Where along this road to perfection can we find a place of health? David O. McKay said something that may be helpful,*" Be tough on yourself but tender with others. "* The great things that have been done in all generations of time have been accomplished by the idealist. Where can we look for an eventual peaceful reign but with those who strive for perfection? Where can we fit in all this seeking for perfection? Are we a help or a hindrance to the progress of mankind? Somewhere, the wisdom of reality must temper idealism into love; Godlike love. Deep, real love often takes a lifetime to develop. It can bring with it the calm, peaceful, harmonious beauty of the well mellowed age. When this wisdom is never learned, if patience and true love is never found, there can be no peace of soul, only the tormented pain that accompanies the unaccepted reality that life and people are not perfect. In this way, the idealist, for all his striving, has missed the mark he set so high, and his punishment is self-destruction. What a waste! If we could even vaguely see the faults of others enough to recognize those poor characteristics that we would not want to make a part of ourselves, we would then make a beginning. It is a sorry fact that the whole life of some people is a waste, except that they serve as a bad example to others. We could also become so trusting of others as to set up a trap for the weak man's dishonesty, thus contributing to their downfall. It would help if we could see and be aware without hate, yet still never give anyone a chance to cheat or steal from us. The words of Christ from the New Testament give us some good advice, *"Be wise as serpents, yet harmless as doves."*

The choices we make can also make us weak and cause us to be ill. Constantly making wrong choices, and often for the wrong reasons, being rebellious and stubborn can cause illness. A person who must have his own way, no matter what, right or wrong, a person who by choice will eat the wrong food, consume alcohol, and smoked tobacco, even if it kills them, is also prone to illness. A person who is indecisive, weak-willed and unable to change even when a better way is known, is susceptible to illness. There are many parents, had they known, would have fed their children much better, but because they did not their child developed weaknesses, chronic disease, and a taste for many of the wrong foods. There are those people who have used drugs, who have learned a better way, who wish they had never allowed the destructive drug to enter their bodies; but the damage has been done. The drugs that still remain in the body can be removed with herbs and mild food, but often the damage they have done can never be repaired.

Environmental weaknesses may also cause illness. Take a child, for example, who is artistic, sensitive, or mechanical, and is not able to express his own personality because one of his parents may have different personality traits and is not able to understand. People we love who are different from ourselves have a way of giving us some polish. J.M. Gibby said, *"When life becomes a grind remember it is only a test to see whether you'll come out broken or polished."* Often the people in our own families help to shape and grind our personalities. At times, those we love the most, can also be our destroyers. Oliver Wendell Holmes spoke of the keys to the heart when he said, *"There is almost always at least one key to this side door. This is carried for years hidden in a mother's bosom. Fathers, brothers, sisters, and friends, often, but by no means so universally, have DUPLICATES OF IT. The wedding ring conveys a right to one; alas if none is given with it."*

Speaking further about the keys to the heart he says, *"Be very careful to whom you trust one of these keys of the side door. The fact of possessing one renders those even who are dear to you very terrible at times. You can keep the world out from your front door, or receive visitors only when you're ready for them; but those of your own flesh and blood, or of certain grades of intimacy, can come in at the side door, if they will, at any hour and in any mood. Some of them have a scale of your whole nervous system and can play all the gamut of your sensibilities in semi tones – touching the naked nerve pulses as a pianist strikes the keys of his instrument. I am satisfied that there are as many great masters of this nerve playing as Vieuxtemps or Thalberg in their lines of performance. Married life is the school in which the most accomplished artists in this department are found."* Too many times we give someone the keys to the door of our heart in marriage; then there is a duplicate of a partner's personality in a child.

The wrong kind of marriage can lead to illness, such as one partner who exercises too much control on a spouse, not allowing the other to express himself or choose for himself, even in diet. There are times when one partner insists inadvertently on killing the other. I knew a man who was given up to die of cancer, who went for help to a health resort. After receiving all the information on diet, returned home only to have his wife say, *"If you are going to eat all that rabbit food you will have to fix it yourself."* The man is now dead this often happens when one partner sees the truth on natural methods of healing and the other partner stubbornly refuses to allow him to do it, thus contributing to the demise of his loved one.

A lack of love or fidelity in marriage can cause an emotional trauma that can lead to physical weakness and even death. People who live together and cannot resolve their problems, physical or personal, often fall ill. There are times when one partner wants an entirely different lifestyle than the other party, causing constant conflict. If a person chooses to remain, he must bring himself into harmony with his partner in order to be well. We must be equally balanced socially, intellectually, spiritually, and physically in order to be well. Many a great genius has hardly found time to eat. The imbalanced life of the professor in being intellectual has caused the jokes about absent-minded professors, or we see the beautiful physical body exercised to the limit, walking around on display with an empty head on its shoulders, or there is the social outcast who never learns to relate to his fellow creatures. There have been some who become so involved in spiritual matters that they wish they were dead, often neglecting the necessities and essentials of daily living, not recognizing that all these things are also relative to health and happiness.

A person who is not making progress lacks achievement. He is an individual that is suffering from an environmental weakness that can cause much illness. War, famine, pollutants in the air and water, and a harshness of the environment – too much sun, heat, etc. – cause us to be weak or ill.

There are those who do not even seem to know when or how to rest or relax – they just go and go until they drop, because of the many demands of a fast-moving society. Sooner or later these externally or internally caused weaknesses in character or our surroundings show up on the iris of the eye in relation to the damage they have done in our being. We have heard a great deal in the past few years about the power of positive thought. The average person is fairly well converted to the belief that if we want anything we must think positively. At times the mind may be sick because the body is sick. At other times the body becomes ill from negative thoughts, sometimes a little of both. Constant fear of cancer because a parent died of the disease will eventually draw it to you like a magnet. Job said, "*For the thing which I greatly feared is come upon me, and that which I was afraid of is come unto me." Job 3:25*

CHAPTER 2

TEXTURE

The density in almost anything determines its strength. It is no different with the human body. We are not born equal. We each have varying degrees of density. Some bodies are loose and flabby and others are solidly packed. We find the same density in wood, for example. Pine or balsa would be easily broken if a hammer were used on it. A solid wood like walnut would not be so easily destroyed.

Normal weight charts for various ages, heights, and frames, cannot be an exact norm simply because some people are more solid, and therefore weigh more. The person who has a fine texture is always solidly packed, until he begins to grow old. As the body softens and becomes more fragile, the close, fine texture of a good inherent body remains on the iris, but as the good inherent body begins to age, the eyes begin to look watery, which is really what is happening inside the body. After death, the body is not entirely eaten by worms – it merely turns to water, and with the exception of the bones, runs away. The more watery the eyes appear, the more watery the body is becoming inside – an almost glassy appearance. Judgment of the density of the body by the texture of the eye is the beginning of correct analysis. They correct determination of healing begins with texture. When the texture is fine, even though many spots may appear or many nerve rings may register on the iris, the fine textured type of body will heal more quickly when given the correct diet and herbs than one with loose texture or lesions.

Many people have asked me how long it takes to change negative markings on the iris. My answer is always the same, "Unless I could follow you around and make sure you take your herbs and vitamins and stay on a cleansing diet I could not say." If a close accurate data to determine the inherent strength or weakness showing the person's ability to heal were kept, as diet was monitored, an accurate judgment as to the time factor could be found. However, to give an overall statement of average fact concerning iridology analysis it requires approximately 3 months of consistent mild food, herbs and vitamins to make any significant change in the iris. The other factor is the ability to throw off waste (inherent body) or what I call vitality. Some people make extremely rapid changes in three months while others make slow progress. The two key factors to observe in the iris are texture and focus. When texture is fine but focuses flat, healing will be at a little slower. When glands are out of balance, healing will be slower, so glands must be the first concern to bring into balance with herbs and diet. If parasite lines or radiation lines appear on the iris, even under the best circumstances, such as fine texture and clear sharp focus, the body will not heal well until the parasites have been killed with herbs. This is why Dr. Jensen noted that when the radii solaris spokes or radiation lines showed on the iris, it would be difficult to heal that part of the body. Consequently, glands and parasites would be of the utmost importance to the time factor in healing.

If a person has inherently poor texture it is not always possible to make a change. In order to survive and remain well, he must live a more healthy life than those having a finer texture.

CHAPTER 3

FOCUS LINES

Sometimes it may be noted in an older person whose texture is excellent that the lines of the eyes have become flat rather than sharply in focus. This indicates the body had good inherent health but is growing old. On the other hand, a young person may have sharp focus but loose texture. He may be stronger at the time than the older person, even though he may be inherently weaker. His body will not last as long as the older person, whose body has had a finer texture. A young person could also have a flat focus and a fine texture merely showing weakness. When a young person has a flat focus and a loose texture, the weakness is compounded. The first thing we look for is inherent strength or texture, then focus.

Focus lines can be changed in many cases by eating more live foods, especially in old age. When the old go to a soft diet and eat fewer raw foods, dark chronic color is increased. When many raw juices are added to their diet, the strength will increase and focus will sharpen where focus is already flat, showing weakness. More raw food, vitamins, and minerals will sharpen the focus, increasing endurance and strength.

CHAPTER 4

EYE COLOR

Dr. Bernard Jensen writes mainly about blue and brown eyes. He mentions a study by the United States Marine Corps done on recruits that noted that blue-eyed recruits make better rifle shots. Of a group of 1200 recruits 66% were blue-eyed. Dr. Jensen further notes that Lieutenant Colonel R.W. Peared of the Los Angeles recruiting office said a large percentage who were good rifle shots had blue eyes. Discussing eye color and longevity, Dr. Jensen notes that there is no evidence that eye color blue or brown has much to do with longevity and that consideration might be given to other eye colors, hazel, gray, etc., as normal. He also observed that eye colors that appear at first glance to be one color are actually, on closer observation under magnification, another.

There has been an ongoing controversy about eye color among iridologists, so I wish to make my position clear on the subject of eye color. There are brown eyes, black eyes, blue eyes, gray eyes, lavender or violet eyes, green eyes, hazel eyes, and two-tone eyes, or even one blue eye and one brown eye. Any or all of these can be normal. From my observation of 40 years of looking into eyes of all races, young and old, and watching the healing process that follows use of nature's rules of healing, it is my opinion that brown eyed people have generally a finer textured iris, showing stronger inherent body's than the other colors, as a general rule. Perhaps they have required more inherent strength to endure the poverty and lack of proper nutrition into which the dark skin and dark eyed people are often born. The colors then following sequence from blue, hazel, green, lavender or violet, to gray as to inherent strength, or beginning genetic overall health. In other words, a person may be able to change all the negative markings of deterioration and never be able to change a green to a blue because it is the color the eye is supposed to be. This is much like cleaning all of the deterioration color out of a shadow weakness area, where the shadow remains, showing that the weakness area is clear but the weakness remains. In a similar way the color remains as natural with the individuals entire body make up. There is a great difference, however, in a hazel eye which is a natural hazel, and a chronic brown showing around the color area of the blue or other light colored eye. When the brown color is evenly distributed from the pupil outward it is a normal hazel eye and no amount of cleansing the colon of the body is going to change the hazel color. True deterioration is beginning from yellow to light brown. Then as it proceeds down to lower layers it is easily distinguishable in the various individual areas. A hazel eye will also extend the brown color out beyond the hazel color and autonomic wreath. There are also occasions when a person has a blue eye which is partially brown. Again it will follow out from the pupil in a smooth, even way, and it is possible that no deterioration is then in the brown area. When deterioration does begin it can easily be seen in the same way as a fully brown eye.

CHAPTER 5

HEART

After determining weakness or strength and color, the next thing we look at is the heart. There should be no markings of any kind showing on the iris in the heart area, unless there is something wrong with the heart.

As far back as 1964 cardiovascular diseases annually killed 921,000 people in the United States. (When the prophets have said in the last days that men's hearts would fail them, it appears that we are living up to expectations.) There are several chief types of heart conditions:

    a) Arteriosclerosis: hardening of the arteries, resulting in high blood pressure.

    b) Hypertension: causing prolonged constriction of vessels and arteries, resulting in high blood pressure.

    c) Rheumatic heart: caused by an acute inflammation resulting in damage to or having an adverse effect on muscles and valves.

    d) Congenital heart: born with diseased or imperfect heart, unable to perform correctly.

e) Mitral stenosis: hardening or narrowing of valve between left atrium and left ventricle, can be congenital or caused by calcium buildup. Hardening of the arteries is caused by scar tissue from surgery, infection, fatty material (cholesterol) or calcium lining the artery walls, causing the opening to become smaller. This causes pressure to build – like putting a nozzle on a hose – increasing the force at which it moves in the arteries. This force may cause a break in the heart or the brain as in a stroke. Calcium salt deposits along the artery walls in rough places causes a hardness and the inability of the artery to flex and perform normal peristaltic action. Hardening of the arteries causes several illnesses, including heart attacks: normally smooth artery linings become rough and narrow because of patchy deposits which interfere with the flow of blood. The rough surface, plus the sluggishness of the blood as it moves through too narrow a channel, sometimes causes a clot, called THROMBOSIS. It may block an artery altogether. Sometimes clots break away from the spot where they form and are carried to other parts of the body in the blood stream. The moving clot is called an EMBOLUS. The coronary arteries that nourish the heart muscle itself are more frequently affected by arterial hardening than any other. Hardening of these arteries causes a decrease in heart muscle blood supply and may cause the chest pains known as ANGINA PECTORIS. Coronary thrombosis is the term used when heart attacks occur where a clot forms and occludes or blocks one of the two coronary arteries that supply nourishment to the heart.

A bowed out, open or closed lesion with only a darker shade than the color of the eye may show on the heart area, indicating organic heart weakness. A brown spot in a lesion or a brown spot in the area of the heart shows deterioration of the heart. Deterioration or cardiac damage shows brown on lesions in an elliptical formation. When there is a splitting separation in the autonomic wreath at 90° on the left iris this shows a structural or organic weakness of the heart. When there is a pathological disturbance of the aorta, the autonomic nerve wreath seems to separate immediately above the heart area. A thickening of the autonomic nerve wreath at the heart area indicates a tension or spasticity of the heart, neurogenic in origin. If there is an incursion of the autonomic wreath towards the pupil at the heart area, disturbances in cardiac functions would again be of a neurogenic origin. A distention of the colon with an incursion out into the heart area indicates that cardiac disturbances will often result because of gas pockets or impactions in the colon. This causes fibrillation or irregular heart, resulting in possible heart failure.

Often there will be no cholesterol showing in the eye, yet the person still has a heart attack. In this case it would be of a neurogenic nature, causing a spastic condition of the heart due to overwork, too much stress, or nervousness. At this time the autonomic wreath would show this spasticity by an incursion toward the pupil at the heart area of the iris, 90° in the left eye.

With the implantation into a human of an artificial heart, interesting new prospects have evolved. The scriptures indicated many centuries ago that you should not put new wine into old bottles. Science has now proven what mechanics have always known about putting new parts into old cars. The main truths that medical science has not understood, with all their technical knowledge, is how the body feeds and eliminates. When after surgery a person is put on a fasting glucose IV, the body automatically begins its toxication process and pneumonia is usually the result. How seriously ill the patient becomes is dependent upon how toxic his or her body was at the time of the surgery. Since doctors know little about nutrition and less about correct body metabolism or what happens when the body fasts, they can only treat the post surgery infections as they occur. If a person has to have major surgery, they would have fewer problems and faster healing if they were prepared and their body cleansed prior to surgery.

The heart is a muscular organ that is hollow with a series of chambers and valves, inlets and outlets, through which blood enters and exits. This is brought about by the muscle contracting and dilating. The heart is located in zone 3 on the left iris between 73° and 93°.

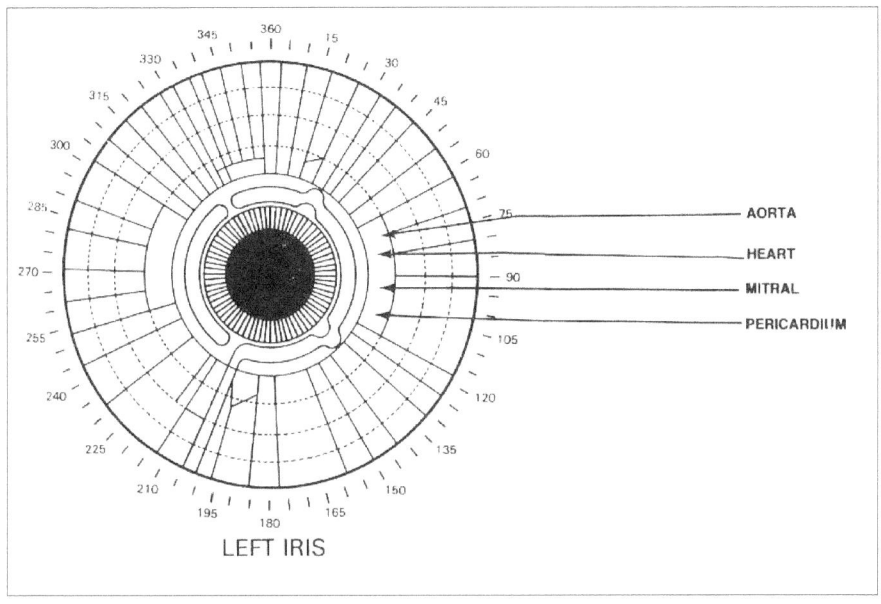

LEFT IRIS

The aorta is located in zone 3 at 60° to 75° on the left iris. The aorta is the main artery of the body. It carries blood from the left ventricle of the heart to all of the organs of the body except the lungs. It also carries blood to the other arteries that supply the body parts with blood.

The mitral valve is the valve between the left ventricle and left auricle of the heart. It is located on the left iris in zone 3 between 93° and 105°.

The pericardium is a thin membrane enclosing the heart and the origin of the great blood vessels. The pericardium is found only on the left iris just below the heart in zone 3 between 105° and 115°.

The pulmonary valve is the valve of the heart that allows blood into the pulmonary artery that goes to the lungs. It shows on the left iris in zone 3 between 73° and 93°.

Cleaning the colon and the entire body usually relieves the burden on the heart, but too much toxic waste moving too fast, pumping through the heart as the body expels the waste, can cause more damage - like taking a shot of deadly poison. People with heart problems must move slowly, eliminating with mild foods and cleansing herbs, and must not try to fast or go on fruit alone. Herbs such as saffron and dandelion that cancel out poison may be used. The heart herbs such as hawthorn (to strengthen the heart muscle), and vitamin E, may be taken. One of the most deadly poisons which can injure the heart in the process of elimination is uric acid. Where kidneys are not properly carrying off the waste, dandelion and saffron and vitamin C have a way of neutralizing this uric acid. Other kidney herbs help to activate the kidneys to a better function. Potassium gluconate and celery juice also help to pull off fluid. Where the kidneys will not respond to such methods, the bowel must be forced to evacuate to a fluid state with highly laxative herbs. This temporarily takes the burden off the kidneys and causes waste to flush out rather than circulate through the heart. In such a case, potassium gluconate should be added to the diet in order to maintain the muscle tone of the heart and other muscles of the body.

Pathologically related signs: albumin, adrenal glands, arm, axilla, esophagus, eyes, foot, gallbladder, hand, liver, lungs, ribs, sternum, urethra, and uric acid.

CHAPTER 6

THE BRAIN

 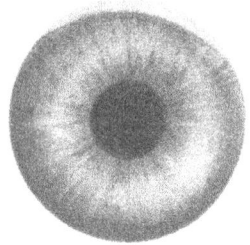

Arcus Senilis

The brain is a mass of nerve tissue located in the skull. It is the main part of the nervous system. It is made out of white matter (the inner mass of nerve fibers), and gray matter (the outer cortex of nerve cells). The brain is composed of the cerebrum, the cerebellum, the pons, and the medulla oblongata. The brain shows on the iris of both eyes from 330° to 30°. The individual parts and functions of the brain are listed separately.

BRAIN

Chronic brown in the head area of the iris is an indication of accumulating toxic waste in the head. Looking at a person's iris where brown deterioration shows as if it were superimposed upon the top of the iris color would probably indicate that this person seldom or never has a cold.

The entire brain is subject to accumulation of toxic waste, as is the entire head and neck. It can therefore be subject to tumors. The brain may be injured from a high fever or lack of oxygen. Certain infections can cause damage to the brain or the spinal cord. This is called ENCEPHALITIS, while infections of meninges or covering of the brain is called MENINGITIS. Inflammation of the roots that emanate from the spinal cord and brain are called RADICULITIS, while inflammation of the nerves is called NEURITIS. Shingles (herpes zoster) is associated with neuritis. Inflammation is always seen as white in the iris in the area affected. Multiple sclerosis attacks the brain and spinal cord, causing deterioration in both.

The brain is encased in a rigid inflexible bond called the skull, where there is virtually no room for expansion. Therefore any swelling, tumors, or hemorrhage exerts pressure on the brain and can cause blindness, convulsions, headache, paralysis, or vomiting. Tumors near the skull can be surgically removed, but when tumors are deep-seated they cannot be entirely removed without causing more problems.

Concussion or severe brain injuries with hemorrhage and swelling can lead to death

Lou Gehrig's disease, in contrast to multiple sclerosis, localizes on bundles of motor nerves in the brain and spinal cord causing slow, progressive paralysis (atrophy).

Demyelinating disease causes degeneration or disappearance of myelin or the insulation around the nerves. It is another brain disease much like stripping away the insulation from an electrical wire. Nerve fibers so affected lose their power to conduct messages to the brain.

Injury or surgery would register immediately as white in the area of the head where the injury had occurred, showing in that given area. When permanent damage has taken place, a gradual process changes the white to brown to black, according to the extent of the injury or surgery.

Much research has been done lately on the involvement of the brain in the healing process. Some of this work has been done by medical scientists, some by clinical psychologists, in determining the role the brain takes in helping the body to heal.

For years the medical professions looked on the brain as only a sophisticated computing and regulating organ. With the advent of the chemical revolution in the 70s, these thoughts have changed radically. The first big discovery was that the brain produces two types of chemicals called endorphins and enkephalins. The chemical endorphin combats pain, the other, enkephalin, is produced to alleviate stress. Since these first two were studied, a variety of chemicals and hormones have been discovered that affect our appetite, blood pressure, sex drive, and so on. It is very clear that the brain is connected to a lot more than just our thought and involuntary responses.

Several case studies and observations have been done that give us a glimpse into the amazing ability the brain has. One case in particular told of a farmer in Colorado who was suddenly subjected to the loss of his two young children who were killed in an automobile accident. Prior to this he had not been prone to sickness; after the accident he suddenly became ill. He slept a lot and lost his appetite. A year and a half later it was discovered that he had bone cancer. He underwent chemotherapy, but it only made him feel worse. Later he began seeing a psychologist and talked about his feelings. It was remarkable: his cancer went into remission. Today he is working on his farm in Colorado. Scientists are quick to say that there are a number of reasons that the cancer might have gone into remission, but none are discounting the fact that his mind might have had something to do with his healing. The opposite of the story happened to a lady in New York. After developing tuberculosis and taking the standard medical treatment, she was partially cured, and the disease went into remission. The woman, herself a pianist, attended a piano concert, realizing that she could not play the piano any longer, she became despondent and within two weeks was dead from the tuberculosis.

Dr. Hans Selye, a Nobel laureate and author of almost 40 books on stress, has come to the conclusion that peaceful thought releases beneficial hormones, while angry thoughts release harmful hormones. Cortisone is a tissue tranquilizer while adrenaline causes aggression. All of this leads us to the conclusion that if we become ill it would be a good idea to think positive thoughts about becoming cured rather than to have a negative attitude that most of us have.

Some of the interesting things that have been learned to help the brain are gotu kola for memory, alfalfa for calcium, and other related minerals, calcium gluconate and calcium lactate for helping circulation to the brain, inversion therapy, exercise and cayenne. More negative ions in the environment, licorice for narcolepsy (wanting to sleep all the time), nervine herbs and vitamin B complex and calcium for nerves will also assist. Lecithin can be used for more brain power, lady slipper for serious brain damage. There are also cleansing formulas for tumors, along with a mild food diet. High doses of vitamin C relieves congestion in the head.

Pathologically related signs: any part of the body may be related.

CEREBELLUM

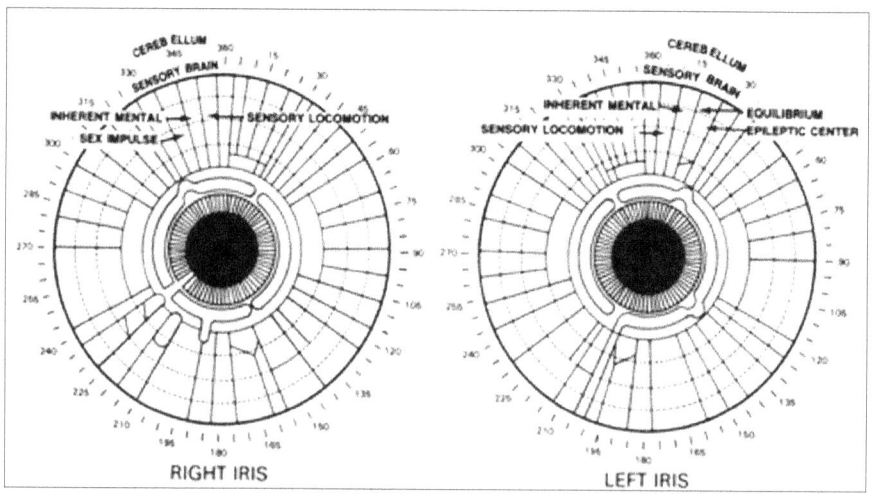

RIGHT IRIS   LEFT IRIS

The cerebellum is the part of the brain below and behind the cerebrum. It is the portion of the brain regarded as the center for coordinating the muscle movement of the body. On the iris on the left eye it shows on most of the area in zones 3, 4, and 5 between 360° and 30°. On the right Iris it is in the same zones, only between 330° and 360°.

Sensory brain

The cerebellum is involved in the control of skeletal muscles and coordination of voluntary muscle movement. On the chart, the sensory areas are designated as follows: sensory locomotion, inherent mental (IQ), sex impulse, perversion, (continual inflammation in the perversion area indicates overstimulation of the sex organs, while chronic markings indicate coldness, lack of stimulation, or frigidity), medulla. Involuntary activity comes from the brain. Medulla oblongata is the enlarged portion of the spinal cord or top of the spinal cord. The medulla coordinates all muscle movements and respiration. If it is damaged in polio, breathing muscles become paralyzed. That is the reason for an iron lung. The medulla acts like a relay or reflex center and connects with higher brain centers, having to do with swallowing, breathing, heartbeat, vomiting, sneezing, sweating, and salivation. How far reaching, then, would an inflammation of the medulla be? Sometimes when it may be difficult to detect the above problems, check the medulla area of the iris. If there are brown or black markings on the iris medulla next to the autonomic wreath, or a split in the autonomic wreath at the medulla section, there is probably interference in the cerebrospinal fluid which bathes the brain, the spinal cord and the choroid plexus itself (which regulates the fluid). Sometimes the area is damaged in a fall, whiplash, or polio. The choroid plexuses are responsible for secreting correct pressure. When this constant pressure is normal, it equals about 175mm of water. If the pressure falls below normal all exocrine and endocrine glands become involved. It has finally been discovered that the choroid plexus secretes a hormone which regulates the spinal fluid. If it drops below the given amount, the hormone activates the secretion of fluid. When animal choroid plexus preparations were used by Dr. R.M. McLain, problems involving spinal fluids were overcome.

The epileptic center is that part of the cerebellum that regulates muscles. The epileptic center is located in zones 4 and 5 on the left iris and almost 25°.

Equilibrium is controlled by the cerebellum. Equilibrium is a state of balance between equal and opposing forces. Equilibrium shows on the iris of the left eye between 18° and 23° in part of zone 3 and in zones 4 and 5.

The inherent mental section of the cerebellum is that part of the brain that deals with the involuntary responses or our mind to body control. It is also our thirst and hunger center. The inherent mental section is located on the left iris between 13° and 18°, on the right iris between 345° and 350° on both eyes in zone 3, 4, and 5.

Sensory locomotion is that part of the brain that controls the major muscles and coordination. It controls the ability to move around. It is located in the cerebellum area of the iris; on the left iris it is found between 3° and 10°, on the right iris between 350° and 357°, on both eyes in zones 3, 4, and 5.

The sex impulse area of the cerebellum is the area that controls the normal desire to have routine sex. If there are problems in this area it can lead to sex perversion or the deviation from normal sexual desires and practices. Both of these areas are located on the right iris between 335° and 345° in zones 4 and 5.

Pathologically related signs: any or all of the glandular diseases, exocrine or endocrine could begin with damage to this area of the body. Check the medulla, dry brain, headache, paralysis, feet, legs, respiratory conditions, circulatory ailments.

CEREBRUM

The cerebrum is the main part of the brain uppermost in the skull. It consists of two equal hemispheres and is the largest part of the brain. It is believed to control voluntary and conscious processes. It is in zones 3, 4, and 5, between 330° and 360° on the left iris and between 360° and 30° on the right iris.

The cerebrum or motor brain is divided into four sections on the iris chart. These are five sense areas, an area for ego pressure, an area for acquired mental speech (ability to communicate), mental ability (learning, reasoning, logic, ability to concentrate, memory, judgment, choice, intelligence, and the emotions), as well as voluntary muscular activities. It is the seat of consciousness.

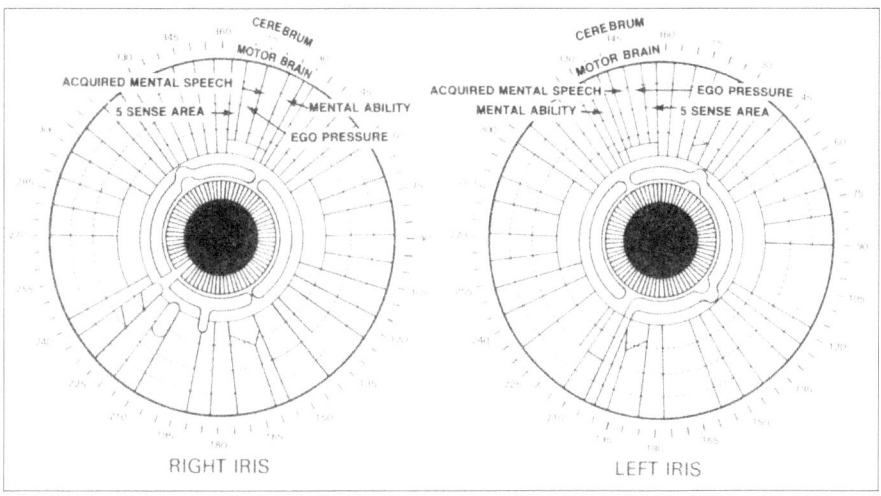

RIGHT IRIS   LEFT IRIS

If the brain is damaged in any way or lacking organically, that is one thing, but it is still another when mental abilities are changed because of a person's lifestyle. Taking drugs, living on a nutritionally poor diet, or driving the body to its absolute limit, causing sight or hearing loss would not be the fault of the brain itself. God has given man his free agency with the exception that he continually stands at the point of decision. He must choose. That is the only thing man is forced to do and choose he must – each second, each hour of the day. The choices he makes regarding his diet can make or break his brain, which then affects every other part of the body. Ego pressure is also important because it deals with individual personality. How each individual response to a given problem or set of problems determines many things regarding health or sickness. A person who is insecure and feels incompetent but does not want anyone to know he is frustrated where his ego is concerned, is often the loud blowhard, braggart type in an attempt to bolster his ego. This type of personality is a prime subject for stroke since the self-imposed stress factor becomes too great. Watch the ego pressure area in this type of individual. After inspection of the ego pressure area, observed directly above the iris on the SCLERA or white of the eye. If the area has a shattered appearance it indicates a possible stroke, high blood pressure, or severe mental disturbance. Check blood pressure. If it is low – with shattered appearance on sclera it indicates serious mental disturbance. If the blood pressure is high, showing the same way and remains high, a stroke is imminent. It is interesting that high blood pressure can also be a result of a toxic bowel condition, and when this is the case, the right side of the body is usually affected. When workload and stress, personal or otherwise, is the cause of a stroke the left side is usually affected. There is a very real connection between the glands and stress (see ADRENAL). There is also a definite connection between the bowel and the brain.

Acquired mental speech on the right iris is located in the cerebrum or motor area of the brain, located between 15° and about 23°. On the left iris the motor part of the brain is located between 340° and 347°.

The inferior frontal gyrus portion of the cerebrum in right-handed persons is more developed on the left side, the opposite on left-handed persons. This area is known as Broca's speech area. Damage to this area results in the inability of physically normal vocal cords to articulate speech.

Ego pressure is that part of the body that regulates the body's response to emotional problems, or to put it in other words, how emotions affect our heart rate, glands, and emotional body temperature. These are located on the left iris between 345° and 350°, on the right iris between 10° and 15°, in both eyes in part of zone 3 and all of zones 4 and 5.

Mental ability is the ability to use thought processes to reason, speak, remember, perceive depth, etc. It is located in the cerebrum. The mental ability area of the brain is located on the iris of the left eye between 330° and 335°, on the right iris between 20° and 27° and in part of zone 3 and zones 4 and 5.

The five sense area of the cerebrum is the area that regulates our ability to perceive things that we see, touch, hear, taste, and smell. This area is located on the left iris between 350° and 335°, on the right iris between 5° and 10°, in part of zone 3 and zones 4 and 5.

Speech in the vocal expression in the communicating of thoughts. It is found in the cerebrum area of the brain. The speech area is located on the left iris between 335° and 340°, in part of zone 3 and zones 4 and 5.

Pathologically related signs: senses, ego, speech, mental ability, and concentration.

MEDULLA OBLONGATA

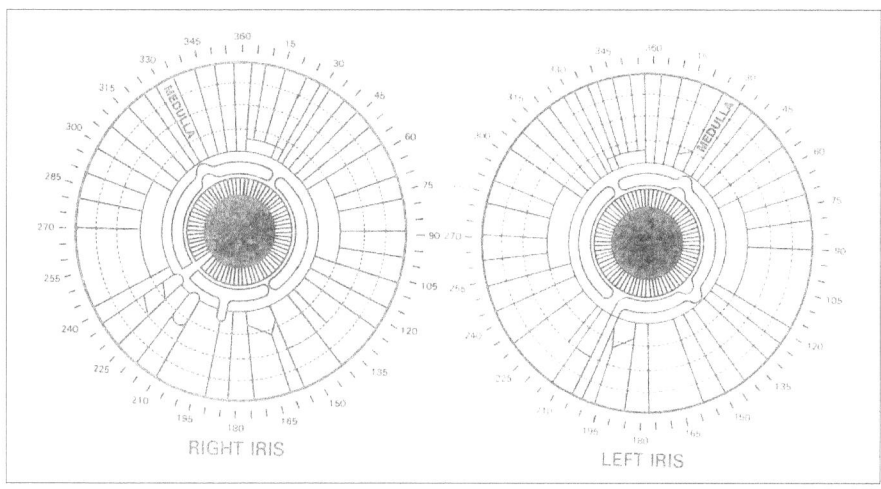

The medulla oblongata is a wide continuation of the spinal cord at the base of the skull forming the lowest part of the brain. It contains vital nerve centers for the control of breathing, circulation, etc. It is located between 25° and 32° on the left iris, on the right iris 327° to 335°.

Whenever there is a spot, lesion, or radii solaris marking close to the autonomic wreath above the transfers colon it indicates that the choroid plexus is having problems.

The choroid plexus maintains cerebrospinal pressure. When pressure is not correct, the endocrine or exocrine can be affected. A fall, whiplash, or polio can cause damage to the choroid plexus. Calcification can also cause damage to the choroid plexus.

The medulla oblongata regulates respiration, heart, swallowing, perspiration, salivation, sneezing, and vomiting. How many far-reaching problems could inflammation of the medulla oblongata cause? It is therefore important to check the area for any acute inflammation.

Animal choroid plexus has been used successfully. However, the herb which acts on the medulla and the choroid as a hormone type herbs is lady slipper.

Pathologically related signs: brain, choroid plexus, endocrine and exocrine glands. (See cerebellum).

CHAPTER 7

CHRONIC COLON-TOXICITY

After analyzing the texture, focus and heart the next in importance would be the bowel and the autonomic wreath. Death begins in the colon. If we had a clogged sewer system in our house we would have more sense than to continue turning on the tap or flushing the toilet, but when it comes to our human sewer system, we do not seem to have a correct conception of its functions. A young Doctor writing for a local newspaper, answering an old woman's inquiry regarding constipation, told her it was normal to go as long as five days to a week without a bowel movement. This is the kind of illogical reasoning which is been taught for too long. After looking in many eyes it will soon be discovered that most chronic deterioration begins in the bowel and along the autonomic wreath. It logically follows, then, that the bowel must be kept clean and emptied as often as food is eaten and digested. If you eat three meals a day, you should have three bowel movements a day. If you eat three meals and have only one movement, you are becoming constipated not only in the bowels, but in the lymphatic system. This has an extreme affect on the brain – (body waste is backing up) a reason for so many headaches and slow thought processes. You will observe that as the body becomes chronically ill, brown splotches or spots begin to appear on the iris of the eye. As the disease process begins a definite change appears in the iris of the eyes. The top or main color of the iris is the natural color of a given eye, blue or brown, etc. When we see inherent weakness either in a shadow or a bowed lesion, the color appears to deepen to a darker shade than the color of the eye. If the body begins to become chronically sick indicating that waste is accumulating in the area where the color changes, the color first changes to a yellow brown then to darker and darker brown to black, which would be complete deterioration down to the bottom layer of the iris. As the correct diet, vitamins, and herbs are followed, the miracle occurs, as the iris color changes back from black to brown to light brown or yellow to white to gone. The changes are simultaneously taking place in the body on a continual cleansing basis of good and bad days. As the toxic waste begins to move out of the cells and lymph of the body into the bloodstream for evacuation, the eyes will whiten on the top of the color of the eye. As waste is being eliminated, the person feels bad. When it cleans out of the body, the person feels better. The way nature heals is through (bad days) elimination and (good days) after waste has been eliminated. White is always a sign of healing, even though a person may be acutely sick, because the waste is on the move, on its way out of the body. When a person is acutely sick as with a cold, flu, pneumonia, measles, mumps, chickenpox, leukemia, and all acute disease, the eye will always be white as though it were coated on top of the color of the eyes – much like a tongue coated white is in acute sickness. An infection or inflammation will also appear white, but will not necessarily be covered over all of the iris. As an acute condition manifests itself, it will be rather white on the top of the color of the eyes, showing only in the area of the infection or inflammation. When white appears between the spoke lines of the iris it indicates that there are parasites holding the inflammation or infection in that given area where it appears. This type is more difficult to overcome than a cold because parasites are involved. Rheumatism or arthritis and lupus often appear in this way before serious deterioration begins and can be mis-analyzed as a general acute condition. Some people have an overlay of white on their eyes continually. This type of person is always weak, tired, and generally feels acutely sick, because his body is always in a state of cleaning (attempting to eliminate waste). This type generally has a fine texture and his body is strong enough to be in a continual state of elimination. He usually feels better immediately upon changing his diet to mild food, thus stopping the intake of mucus forming foods the body has been trying to eliminate. Where people with loose texture do not have the ability to eliminate waste as readily, they begin to store waste in the lymphatic system and cells, causing the body to deteriorate in the given areas of weakness. It has been said that wherever inherent weakness shows on the iris indicating a given part of the body, this is where a person will get sick when they grow older. In other words those are the areas were a body will deteriorate first. When the stage of white is reached, often a healing crisis will purge the remaining waste from the body, and the eye will clear to its normal color.

When any chronic spots or lesions show deterioration, mild food and cleansing herbs should be used until spots are removed and healing is complete. Many times when people feel better they stop and go back to concentrated foods before they have sufficiently cleansed.

A young man at one of the health conventions who claimed to be an iridologists told me he did not believe the eye changed. What good would iridology be to anyone if the iris did not change as the body healed? Different doctors during a person's lifetime would always be treating the same thing if it remained on the iris. He further stated that he had put people on a good diet and given them homeopathic medicines and they were healed, yet the markings in the eye had not changed. My answer was that the person or persons were not healed, or the changes would take place on the iris.

The story is told of a man who had a gold mine and spent thousands of dollars hoping to hit the mother lode. Finally, after many years, and much money, he gave up and sold his mine. The man who bought the mine found the mother lode just 2 feet from where the original owner had stopped digging.

People often make the same mistake with their health and think they can abuse their body as long as they feel all right, not realizing that, *"Death is a gradual process, only its consumption seems sudden". (J.M. Gibby)*

People often return to a bad diet as soon as they begin to improve, not recognizing that the disease is not completely rooted out. The return from sickness to health is a gradual process, and how quickly healing takes place is related to focus and texture. Texture and focus determine the body's ability to heal, showing how much strength and vitality and ability the body has to throw off waste. By the same token, markings can be cleared off the iris where weakness remains and later in life if diet standards are weakened, the problem area becomes toxic again and the markings return.

Good health has to be worked at on a continuing basis, not living good for a while until one feels better and then junking out again. It is therefore important to live while you are alive, and to live well is to be disciplined in all respects with regard to diet, exercise, water, stress, supplements, and rest. It naturally follows that the weakness in focus and texture that is apparent in a person's iris the greater he must work and staying well, or he will simply shorten his own life.

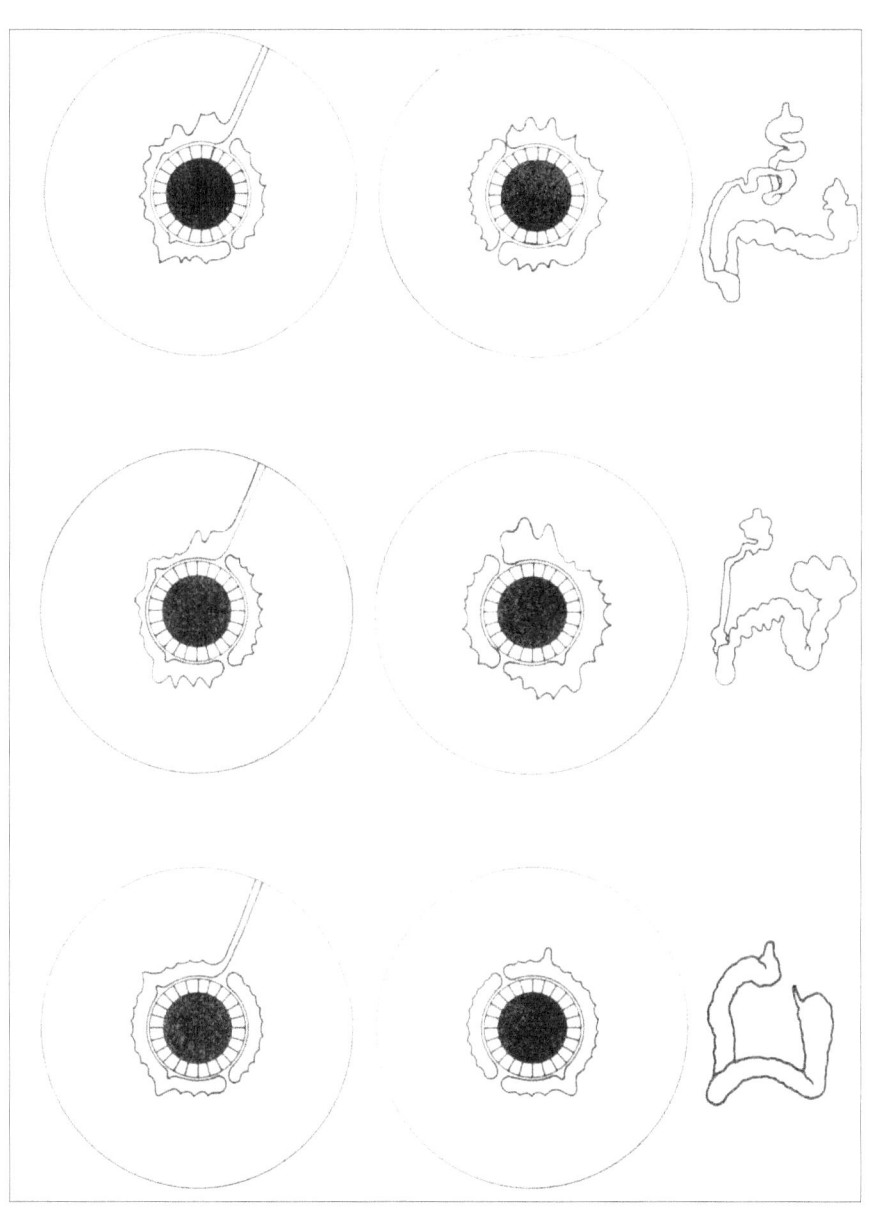

CHAPTER 8

COLON AND STOMACH

The stomach appears on the iris next to the pupil in the first zone. The color appears around the outside of the stomach line with the transverse colon cut in half at the naval. Showing half of the transverse colon on the right eye and half on the left eye above the pupil. The ascending colon appears on the right eye para-limbal region adjacent to the stomach area on the ear side of that eye. The small intestines are in the center para-limbal region of the stomach area on the nose side of each eye. Wherever the colon or small intestines appear in any other shape than shown on the chart – either an incursion or an excursion with a pocket or sharp points in or out, this indicates a distortion in the colon itself. When there is an incursion toward the pupil, it indicates spasticity, a pinching off of the colon, shrunken in that area. An incursion away from the pupil out of the normal second zone indicates a lack of tone or a distention. Often in this distention there will be brown or black ballooned out pockets deterioration, showing the colon to be filled with all manner of toxic, chronic waste, possibly accumulated for years. This waste clings to the pocket walls of the colon, hardens and fills with worms. If there are pinworms involved, many black dots will appear like black pepper on the colon area, if other microscopic parasites are involved, the radii solaris line will seem to project out from the inside of the colon line itself. Some radii lines will seem to project from the pupil out like spokes in a wheel. These dark shape, cut lines will often be confused with darkening lesions in the bowel or stomach.

COLON

RIGHT IRIS   LEFT IRIS

The ascending colon shows only on the right iris, taking up the area just past the stomach line and before the autonomic wreath, starting at about 240° proceeding to 330° in zone 2.

The ascending colon is that part of the large intestine on the right side of the lower abdomen. It starts at the cecum and continues upward until it reaches the right lobe of the liver, where it flexes to the left. It remains at the posterior wall of the abdomen next to the peritoneum.

The anus is located at about 200° to 205° on the left iris. The anus or anal canal is the determining point of the digestive system of the body and the lowest end of the colon.

The vermiform appendix is a long tubular appendage of the colon. It starts at the cecum and may project in any of several directions. On the right iris it is located in zone 1 at 190°.

Pathologically related signs: cecum, groin, liver, and colon.

CECUM

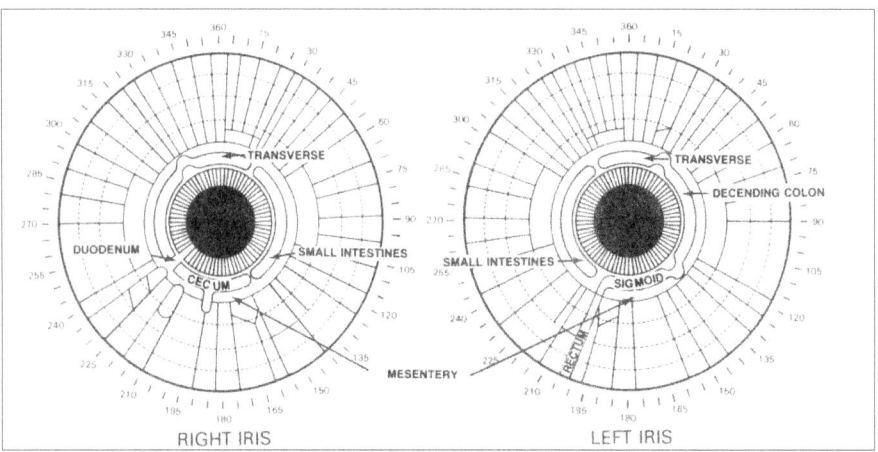

The cecum has been considered by most people who understand natural healing to be the area infested most with worms. More often than not what appears to be an appendicitis attack is in reality only a cecal inflammation. In order to be a true appendicitis attack, the iris will again tell. Note the area of the appendix extends down into the abdominal area of the iris. If acute inflammation (white) is not showing in the abdominal area it is only in the cecum. Many times the appendix has been removed unnecessarily.

The cecum is the blind pouch portion that is the beginning of the large intestine. It is located on the right iris at about 180° in zone 2.

Mild food and cleansing herbs may be used. Psyllium may also be used, as it is with most problems in the digestive system. Colon therapy may also be effective.

Pathologically related signs: colon, small intestines, appendix, spleen, hay fever, thymus gland, pituitary gland, eyes, ears, and congestion in the head area.

The descending colon shows only on the left iris on zone 2, taking up most of that zone from 30° to 135°. The descending colon is that portion of the large intestine on the left side of the lower abdomen. It is connected on the top of the transverse colon; on the bottom to the sigmoid portion of the colon.

The duodenum is the first section of the small intestine that connects the stomach to the small intestine. It is so called because it is about 12 fingers in length. It shows only on the right iris at 227° to 235° in zones 1 and 2.

The mesentery is a membranous fold that attaches various organs to the body wall, especially the peritoneal fold attaching the small intestine to the back abdominal wall. It is found on the left iris at about 165° in zone 2, between the small intestine and the cecum.

The rectum is the last section of the large intestine. It begins at the end of the sigmoid flexure and goes to where the anus begins. It is found on the left iris only, between 200° and 205° in zones 2 through 4.

The sigmoid flexure is the last curving part of the large intestine, ending in the rectum. It shows on the iris of the left eye between 135° and 195° in zone 2.

The small intestines are the narrow, coiled and twisted upper part of the intestines extending from the stomach to the large intestine. The small intestines are identified on the left iris in the second zone from 210° to 330°, on the right iris in the same zone from 30° to 150°.

The transverse colon is that part of the large intestine that crosses from side to side. It is the longest and most movable part of the colon. It passes from right to left. It lies between the upper hip bones just behind the navel. They can be found on the iris of both the left and right eyes between 330° and 30° in zone 2.

In order to change the appearance of a chronic colon on the iris of the eye because of changes taking place in the colon itself, it is often necessary to take colonic irrigation along with the mild food diet and cleansing herbs. The herb psyllium may be taken one or 2 tablespoons a day in water or juice. Psyllium will form a soft bulk attaching itself to the hardened fecal matter in the chronic pockets, pulling off hardened ropelike putrid and rotten waste which may have been there for years. Psyllium will assist in healing torn places, while slippery elm and okra are also healing and soothing to a sore colon. Goldenseal and cayenne are herbs that stop internal bleeding; goldenseal is also antibiotic. The cleansing herbs, along with psyllium, a mild food diet, and some enemas, have been known to bring the colon back to its normal function, which is to carry off most of the body waste. Remember, death begins in the colon. Whenever the bowel is chronically ill, vitamin B_6 added to the diet in the form of acidophilus cultures activates and assists the large and small intestines to accomplish their purposes. Any chronic deterioration on the small intestines is a good indication that food is not being properly assimilated. The absorption of nutrients to be used in the body takes place through the small intestinal walls by means of osmosis into the bloodstream. If these walls are clogged with tumors, toxic waste, cholesterol or hardened oils, the absorption cannot accurately take place no matter how good the diet may be. Chronic deterioration shows on the black spotted area shown on the chart as pey-pat (Peyers patches). Damage could have been done to this area when there was a high fever as a child. This type of person will always have to take more vitamins and minerals in order to maintain health or growth. When some children who do not seem to grow well have their diet improved without changes in the condition, damage to the peyers patches is often found to be the cause. If the area of the small intestines is only chronically brown or black for other reasons, a cleansing of this part of the body becomes the first and most important step in order to regain health. Again, psyllium and a mild food diet is used.

Because waste has no clear way out, close lesions have a more difficult time changing than open lesions. A mild food diet and cleansing herbs are used. Healing lines will appear across lesions as if you were weaving crisscross threads over the lesions. When they appear it indicates that healing is beginning to take place.

Where the transverse colon appears to be nonexistent above the pupil, a prolapsed colon can be found. When the colon is prolapsed, muscle tone must be increased by leg up exercises, lying on a slant board, inversion therapy and taking potassium gluconate. A person with a prolapsed colon or female organs should never do sit-ups. Potassium is the muscle toning mineral and sometimes, in the life of a person who has a prolapsed colon, potassium has been deficient for an extended period of time. Prolapsis usually happens during the growth period of puberty, but not always. Anytime the colon is prolapsed other vital organs are also subject to problems.

Ascending colon

Pathologically related signs: when the ascending colon has impactions of toxic fecal matter the signs are calcium deficiency, general vitamin deficiency, and problems with the thyroid gland, mammary glands, thymus gland, pituitary gland, ears, and tonsils. The person will be subject to asthma, appendicitis, poor digestion, adenoids, hay fever, chronic waste in the head and nasal area, pinworms, hiatal hernia, bronchitis, problems with the cecum, and eyes.

Transverse colon

Pathologically related signs: liver, female organs, prostate, gallbladder, heart, stomach, pylorus, throat, bronchials, esophagus, trachea, sub-maxillary glands, and diaphragm.

Descending colon

When the descending colon is impacted with toxic waste the pathologically related signs are: uterus and prostate, genital glands, rectal fissures, hemorrhoids, bladder problems, testicle problems, kidneys, adrenaline, albumin, pancreas, abdominal wall, groin, peritoneum, and small intestines.

STOMACH

The stomach is a large, sac like organ into which food, passed from the esophagus, is stored and begins the early stages of digestion. The stomach takes up all of the first zone of both the right and left iris.

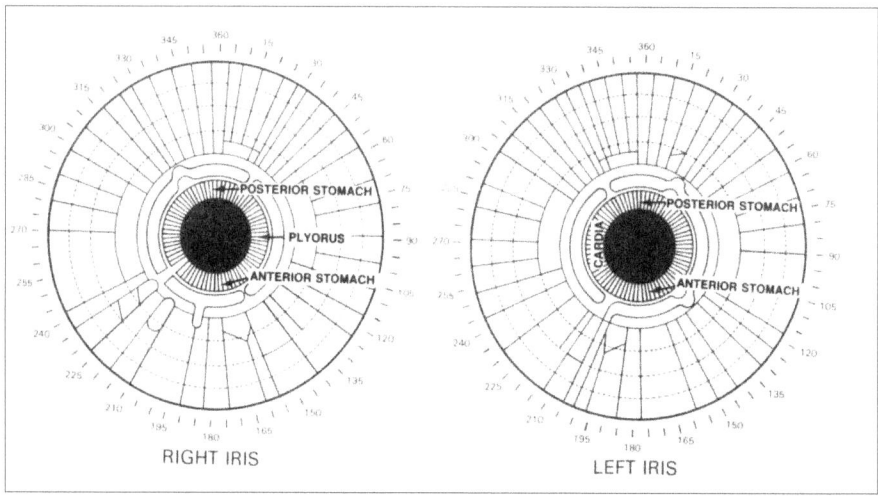

RIGHT IRIS   LEFT IRIS

The most common problem the stomach has is with ulcers. Peptic ulcer is a general term for ulcers that occur in the stomach, but these more commonly occur in the duodenum. The ulcer that occurs in the stomach is the gastric ulcer or one that is positioned in the stomach wall.

A mild food diet has been used effectively to heal ulcers, but a faster, more effective therapy is to use cabbage juice with a fast. Cabbage juice may also be used with a mild food diet and herbs. The herbs to use for an ulcer are okra in a dosage of about two tablets or three capsules before meals, slippery elm about two capsules before meals, comfrey and chickweed teas, and bitter root. The vitamins that have been used are B complex, A, and approximately 2000 mg per day of vitamin C. If acid stomach is caused by adrenaline stress see ADRENAL GLAND.

Parts of the stomach

The anterior stomach, or front portion of the stomach, is also called the lesser curvature of the stomach. On the right and left iris the anterior portion of the stomach shows on the lower portion of zone 1.

The cardia is the upper part of the stomach, more specifically the cardiac glands, the glands that secrete mucus. The Cardia is located on the iris of the left eye at about 270° in zone 1.

The posterior stomach, or the rear portion of the stomach, is also called the greater curvature of the stomach. On the right and left iris both the posterior position of the stomach shows on the upper portion of zone 1.

The pylorus is the opening from the stomach into the duodenum, (the first part of the small intestine). It is found on the right iris only. It is positioned in zone 1 at 90°.

Pathologically related signs: abdominal wall, bile duct, diaphragm, esophagus, gallbladder, liver, and peritoneum.

CHAPTER 9

AUTONOMIC WREATH

The autonomic wreath is next in importance when viewing the iris. It is difficult for the body to heal when the autonomic wreath is chronic in color. When the nervous system of the body is functioning normally, the waste of the body is cleared out more rapidly. When the autonomic wreath or nervous system is well or normal, where there is a condition showing yellow to brown to black, the body heals very slowly, because the autonomic wreath has to do with the sympathetic autonomic nervous system of the entire body. If a radio had corrosion on many of the wires, even if you plugged it in and turned it on, the radio would not play well. The nervous system is a very intricate and vast system; its messages are carried as secretly as conversation on a telephone wire.

Nerve cells look like a drop splashed on a hard surface with tentacles flung out in all directions. The cell body is the central blob, the part sprayed out resembling tree roots are called DENDRITES.

Another long single fiber attached is called and AXON; it ends in a brush like tip. The complete unit is called a neuron. Dendrites accept incoming impulses and carry them toward the cell body. The axon carries impulses away from the cell body. Nerves vary in diameter according to how many axon fibers are bundled together like cables. Each fiber is an extension of a cell body that may lie a great distance away. The sciatica nerve, for instance, runs from the back to the tip of the toes. Most axons are covered by a white fatty material called MYELIN. Myelin is like the rubber insulation used on electrical wires and may serve other purposes.

Billions of neurons are found in the body – some 12 billion in the brain alone. This is fortunate, for medical science says we cannot regenerate nerve cells. A limited amount of nerve repair is possible as long as the cell body remains intact. The neuron functions in such a way that if a nerve is forever cut or injured, the part attached to the cell body remains, but the part beyond withers away. Sometimes a live part can extend itself through the withered component to reach its original destination and restore function. In some cases several nerves can be rejoined by a surgeon, but only when nerve tracts are accessible; unfortunately many are not.

Electricity follows a continuous wire at a speed of 186,000 miles per second; nerve speed impulses travel only 200 miles an hour. This is fast, but not instant. We cannot safely rely on quick reflexes to get out of trouble. It takes about 1/10 of a second for nerve impulses to warn us and another split-second to act on the information, except where extreme fear is involved. On the latter, a shot of adrenaline floods the system. Unfortunately, our fear antenna is only geared to certain reflexes by what has been computed into our brain through or by great parental love and training (reaction to a child's cry, etc.).

Nerve impulses travel in a chain reaction; one neuron triggers the next like a trail of gunpowder that ignites point by point as heat reaches each neuron. This is an electrochemical process which depends on movements of molecules back and forth across membranes of a nerve fiber. The inside of a resting fiber is negatively charged, the outside positively charged. This is caused by the relative abundance of potassium ions in the interior and sodium ions in the exterior. The firing of a neuron changes the permeability of the membranes with an inward flow of sodium and an outward flow of potassium, reversing the electrical charge. Almost instantly, sodium, potassium movements are reversed and so is the electric charge. These alternating movements of molecules across membranes produce currents that propagate a nerve impulse. Reversals occur as frequently as 1,000 times a second; thus, a nerve impulse is a series of tiny electrical breaks which travel over fibers and are boosted from one point to the next by chains of electrochemical relay stations which give local reinforcement of power.

A given stimulus either causes a single neuron to discharge or it does not. Communication between individual neurons is virtually infinite in number since the cells are not physically attached. Such loose connections permit uncountable numbers of switching arrangements. The junction where fine terminal branches of axons come close to dendrites of another neuron is called synapse. There is no direct contact; a synapse is like a spark gap which a nerve impulse must jump across. This jump is helped by a body chemical, acetylcholine, which is essential for nerve impulse transmission. An excess accumulation compels various organs and tissues to run wild, causing a paralysis like effect (like nerve gas) and toxic buildup. We have a natural defensive enzyme called cholinesterase which breaks down acetylcholine as fast as it is formed. A fantastically rapid nerve ending buildup and breakdown of opposing chemicals keeps nerve impulses flowing in good order between synapses.

When too much toxic waste is accumulated, the body must operate rapidly to keep up with this, reminding one of an old-fashioned movie being run too quickly. When this function becomes worn out and fatigued, what happens then? What happens when certain glands do not function because of the lack of certain hormones or because of overwork, causing fatigue of the glands? What happens when calcium, sodium and potassium are not in proper balance? There is no difference whatever between nerve impulses except in frequencies per second. There is not a special kind of nerve impulse for seeing and another for smelling or tasting. If some incredibly mischievous rerouting of nerve pathways should occur, we would perhaps be able to hear a flavor or smell a sunset. Something of this nature arises because of glandular imbalance or growths in nervous tissue which may cause unreal but vividly perceived sensations. These are hallucinations of taste, vision, and indeed, all senses which have no detectable physical basis. This is what drugs do (LSD, liquor, etc.). Could it be that drugs settle in spots where nerves cannot function, causing a rerouting or an obstruction in transmission? Could this be how acupuncture works, using an inorganic needle in these places? Since the electrical system works totally on organic substances it can get clogged, or when placed in certain areas, cause transmission to cease.

How important, then, is the autonomic nerve wreath on the iris? In my opinion, it is of the utmost importance. This area gives an exact accounting of how far the entire nervous system has deteriorated or is healing. White would show an acute condition, and it is interesting to note that when there may be nothing else wrong appearing on the iris and the wreath is white, the body can be in a great deal of pain. The sodium ring and the brown ring around the pupil are considered to be drug rings on the iris, but it is my opinion that when the iris shows globs of orange to brown on the autonomic wreath drugs are involved in the nervous system of the body. It naturally follows, then, that cleansing herbs and mild food clean the body of toxic waste accumulated through the nervous system. The cleansing of other affected parts of the body does not take place until the wreath is clear.

To alleviate problems with the autonomic wreath, the nervine herbs are used to strengthen and heal the nervous system. Vitamin B complex, calcium lactate or gluconate, cleansing formulas and mild food diet may also be used. Cleansing herbs and a mild food diet clean the body of toxic waste accumulated through the nervous system. As this is cleansing, other parts will clean also, but a complete cleansing of other affected parts of the body does not take place until the wreath is clear. In order to further strengthen the nerve activity while cleansing is taking place, vitamin B complex and calcium of a lactate or gluconate type will increase the body's ability to throw off the waste. Whenever there is a break in the wreath, or a week wreath that is hardly showing or even almost nonexistent, the nervine herbs, vitamin B complex and calcium should be used, approximately 6 capsules or six tablets of each daily. When the wreath is white, the whole body is in pain, because the nervous system is in an acute condition of elimination. In this case high doses of vitamin C from 1000 to 2000 mg an hour have been used. A fruit and juice diet, like that used to treat a cold, could be used until the pain subsides or until the white autonomic wreath is changed to just a darker shade than the color of the eye.

CHAPTER 10

NERVE RINGS

Nerve rings appear as a partial or complete line all the way around the iris, and are associated with the autonomic wreath. When the wreath is white either the body is in an acute condition, cleansing or both. Sometimes there will be problems showing in the wreath and no nerve rings, at other times there will be nerve rings and no problems with the wreath. Nerve rings indicate nervousness while problems in the wreath can even indicate a total no-feel situation.

Where many drugs have been used or there is damage to the nervous system itself, the person's body may be either feeling nothing or feeling everything, or even having a hallucination type of condition. At times the damage to the wreath is so pronounced that the synapses cannot be completed in the given areas of obstruction in transmission. This obstruction is exactly pinpointed on the autonomic wreath according to color, from orange to brown to black. A brown color in the rings indicates they have been there a long time. Where the nerve ring crosses the spinal area it can be determined exactly where a chiropractic adjustment will be needed. When the ring follows all the way around the iris in a connected manner, the entire nervous system of the body is affected. When there are three rings connecting all the way around, the subject is usually ready for a complete nervous breakdown. How quickly a breakdown occurs is dependent upon the strength or weakness in texture. There is a more serious condition when rings and wreath are both affected, and paralysis will often appear this way. There will be other things to consider: markings showing a chronic spot or lesion on the medulla in the brain area; markings on the spinal area – thickening of the autonomic wreath, giving the colon and stomach area a three-dimensional or concave appearance. In disabling paralysis there are also markings showing on legs or arm areas.

Where there are chronic nerve rings showing, check the autonomic nerve wreath. When white nerve rings come and go, find out who or what is causing the nervous tension. Change the environment or attitude towards the environment. Vitamin B complex calcium lactate or gluconate, and nervine herbs may be used to alleviate the problem.

It is extremely important to maintain cleanliness of the body tissues, especially the bowel, as elimination is often slowed down to the point where the body deteriorates very rapidly if this essential process is not taken care of. It is also important to feed the nervous system those elements which soothe and strengthen: nervine herbs such as red clover, lobelia, hops, catnip, valerian, chamomile, etc., and vitamins and minerals necessary to feed the nervous system such as B complex and calcium lactate or calcium gluconate. Of course it is also important to remove the cause of stress, if possible. Often a person will not even realize that certain things in his daily life are irritating his nervous system.

Mothers would do well to check their children's eyes for nerve rings, thereby recognizing problems in the child's life. A wise mother could then make an effort to determine the cause of the nervousness. The child may be having problems in school or other emotional stress. If the stress of the child's life is not improvable, the mother could at least give the child sustaining herbs and vitamins to see him through the stress.

CHAPTER 11

GLANDS

The various glands of the body are in trouble when any lesions or spot markings show on a particular gland area. The lines of the eyes normally project out straight from the autonomic wreath to the peripheral line of the iris. Wavy lines indicate glandular imbalance. If there are no markings or lesions showing on any of the glands but the lines are wavy, it is always adrenal imbalance caused from too much stress, a dramatic shock, or a great or extended unsolvable stress.

Dr. E. Hugh Tuckey gave us the valuable information of hydrochloric acid (footnote as found in National Health Federation Bulletin October 1967) for use in digestion. He said that the major role of hydrochloric acid is to digest protein, and if there is too little hydrochloric acid, the stomach does not empty as soon as usual and foods eaten 3 to 4 days earlier and not digested causes putrefaction, causing gas, a belching condition, a burning in the stomach, and a substernal burning just behind the breastbone. He says further that a person with these problems will then take a bicarbonate of soda or other type of antacid to alkalize a stomach that already does not have enough acid, when often the antacid used will be aluminum preparation which he says can cause cancer.

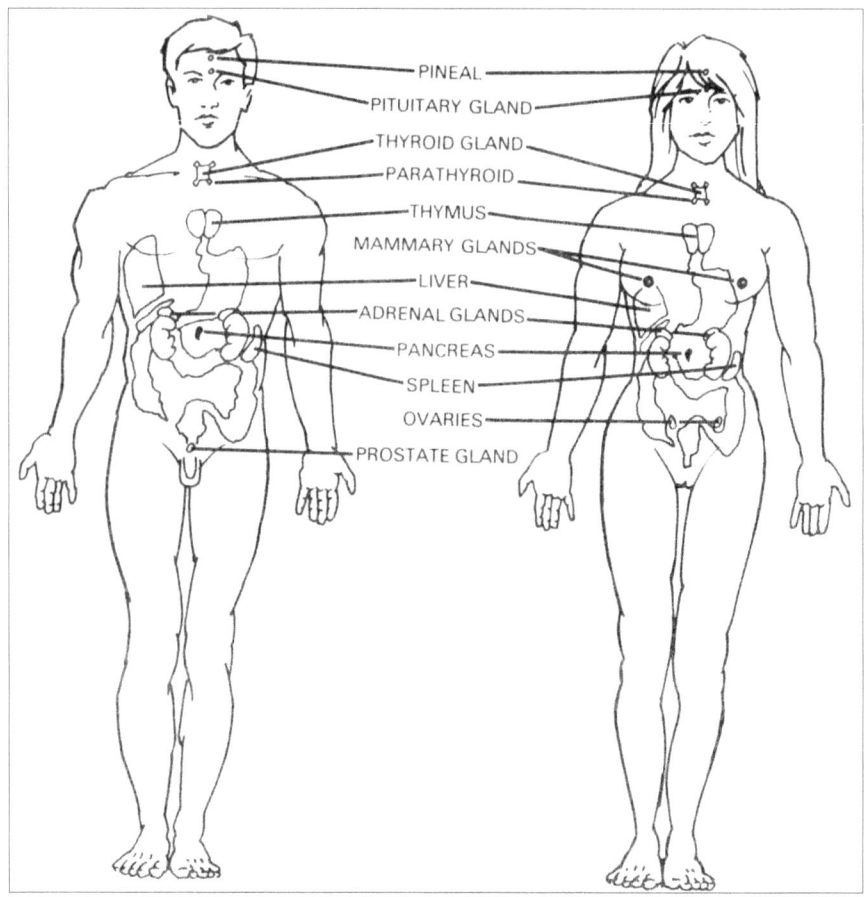

PINEAL
PITUITARY GLAND
THYROID GLAND
PARATHYROID
THYMUS
MAMMARY GLANDS
LIVER
ADRENAL GLANDS
PANCREAS
SPLEEN
OVARIES
PROSTATE GLAND

He states also that in tests, lactic acid shows up in the stomach in these cases, and it does not belong there at all. When the emptying time of the stomach is slowed down due to hypo-achlorhydria, he says we always find a spastic pylorus and we can demonstrate this clinically on 100 times out of 100; we don't have to guess at it. Then he has shown how this spasticity in turn involves the bile duct and pancreas duct. If the pylorus is in a state of spasm, the duodenum is also in a state of spasm, so a normal amount of bile is not emptying into the small intestines. One of the properties of bile is one of being a bactericide along with promoting the peristalsis of the small intestines. This also causes the liver to become engorged with bile that should be going into the small intestines. The pancreas is also affected, causing a backing up of its secreting substances. The pancreas them becomes enlarged, hard, and extremely tender. We can see that this lack of hydrochloric acid has far-reaching effects involving the stomach, liver, gallbladder, pancreas, assimilation of food, constipation, pancreatitis, and even hepatitis. Dr. Tuckey gave hydrochloric acid to his patients so that people could handle the protein and found that they would have to take these on an indefinite basis unless they were given a pancreatic duodenal substance, then the hydrochloric acid would normalize in 2 to 4 months. Dr. Tuckey was not clear on the cause of the problem but rather thought it could be caused from emotions and the stress of everyday incompatible living conditions. He has given us some very valuable information resulting from 30 years of research. He suggests the use of hydrochloric acid tablets when traveling in countries where there is bad water. These will kill the amoebas in the water and prevent diarrhea discomfort. It is with apprehension that I mentioned his findings, and I wish to add to rather than distract from his work. It is been my discovery that the cause is as he had supposed, and adrenaline cortin hormone which interferes with the production of hydrochloric acid, causing a uric and lactic acid buildup in the stomach. Lactic acid builds in the muscles from exercise and the excess is normally routed back to the liver and changed to glycogen so it can be used again as energy. Seepage through the abdominal wall could result if the liver is clogged in the way he has described and so seeps into the abdominal tissue and into the stomach, causing the burning sensations experienced when lactic acid is present in the stomach.

The diseases that are associated with the adrenal glands are Addison's disease, hyperglycemia, and hypoglycemia. The herbs that act in a similar way to help the adrenals to heal our licorice or wild yam. A good multivitamin is used for the adrenals, along with vitamin B complex, and B6 where the colon is ulcerated. The minerals essential are calcium, fluorine, iron, silicon, phosphorus, sulfur, iodine, and manganese. Medical science uses the drug hydrocortisone, which is known to be harmful when taken over an extended period. Licorice acts like cortisone in that it appears to regulate the hormone production for the adrenals, assisting an individual's ability to undergo stress, emotional and physical. Mild food is essential, along with multivitamins, calcium gluconate or lactate. Saffron is the herb, along with dandelion, that has been used in conjunction with licorice to stop the buildup of uric and lactic acid as well as aid digestion. Where the bowel is ulcerated, psyllium and cleansing formula are used. Tumors in the adrenals require also a cleansing formula and psyllium, and high doses of vitamin C, 3000 to 4000 mg a day. When laxative herbs are taken for extended periods of time, potassium gluconate is then added to the diet, approximately 4 to 9 - 600 mg tablets. A mild food diet is an essential part of making a change in glandular functions.

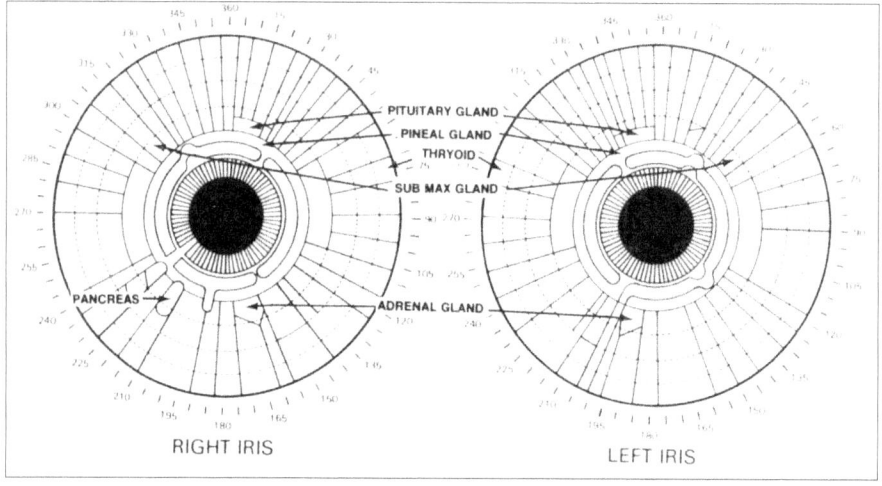

RIGHT IRIS

LEFT IRIS

The adrenal glands are located in the third zone out from the pupil, on the right iris between 155° and 175°, on the left iris between 184° and 175°.

The adrenal glands is made up of two parts. The cortex is the outer zone of the gland and produces the hormone cortin. The inner part of the gland is called the medulla and produces epinephrine (adrenaline). Both of these internal secretions help the body to deal with stress, cortin with every dray stress, adrenaline with high physical and emotional stress, allowing the person to run or fight in an emergency.

Pathologically related signs: lack of muscle tone, heart problems and all other glands can be affected, bowel problems, kidneys, skin pigmentation, mental disorder, confusion, abdominal wall, back, bile duct, breast, jaw, peritoneum, ribs, and uric acid.

The pancreas is a large, elongated gland positioned behind the stomach. This gland produces an external secretion that contains digestive enzymes. Internally it produces insulin glycogen. The pancreas shows on the right iris between 210° in 220° in zone 3.

Diabetes is the disease that is associated with the pancreas. The pancreas produces the hormone insulin. If the pancreas is no longer able to produce insulin then it has to be taken in the drug form. Insulin breaks down sugar and carbohydrates, which the body needs to sustain life. Goldenseal and Juniper berries are nature's insulin and can be substituted for the drug insulin. This changeover is best done slowly by decreasing the amount of insulin and increasing the amount of goldenseal.

One of the primary reasons that a pancreas slows down or stops is the excess use of sucrose or common white sugar, molasses, sorghum, brown or raw sugar. Insulin breaks these sugars down into glucose so that the body can use them. If a person uses too much sucrose in his diet the pancreas becomes overworked and eventually is unable to produce the insulin, resulting in diabetes. Another reason for the malfunction of the pancreas is the accumulation of parasites invading the islands of Langerhans, interfering with the production of insulin. Pumpkin seed, pumpkin seed oil or herbal pumpkin formula may be used to kill any parasites that may be present in the pancreas. These herbs can reverse the disease simply by killing the parasites if no permanent damage has been done to the pancreas (see *To Your Abundant Health).* Herbs, vitamins, and minerals to use in conjunction with goldenseal or juniper berries and vitamin B complex, chlorine, magnesium, potassium, sodium, and calcium.

Pathologically related signs: nerve rings, toxic bowel, fluid buildup, wavy lines on the iris, retina damage, parasites that will show as radii solaris lines (spokes like the spokes of a wheel that show up on the iris when parasites are present). Other pathologically related signs are abdominal wall, ribs, and spleen.

Parathyroid: The herbs used to regulate parathyroid problems are iodine and alfalfa. These two herbs together act as the parathyroid hormones and have regulatory effect on the parathyroid's. A good cleansing formula should be used if tumors are involved. A good multivitamin and mineral supplement is essential. A mild food diet rich in fresh vegetables and fruit is important. Additional calcium gluconate or lactate is also necessary.

It is necessary to determine if any of the other glandular areas are in need of help. Alfalfa and iodine will stop muscle spasms almost immediately.

Pathologically related signs: thyroid, all other glands, bowel problems, kidneys, congestion in the head, fluid retention, muscle spasms, convulsions, nervous disorders, atlas and axis vertebrae, breast, jaw, larynx, lens, nose, pharynx and tonsils.

The pineal gland is a small pinecone shaped gland attached to the post part of the third ventricle of the brain. Its function is unknown. It has sometimes been called the spiritual gland. On the left iris it is found next to the pituitary gland in zone 3 between 333° and 343°. On the right iris it is found in the same position between 20° and 27°.

The pituitary gland is a small oval shaped gland that produces secretions that are sent through the blood and lymph to various parts of the body. The pituitary gland is the main gland of the body influencing body growth. On the left iris it is located in zone 3 between 343° and 357°. On the right iris it is located between 3° and 20°.The herb which acts to regulate the pituitary gland is alfalfa. It requires up to 20 or more tablets per day to make changes. Medical science uses a drug called ACTH as the pituitary hormone. People with a problem in the pituitary gland also need to take the minerals: phosphorus, sulfur, manganese, iodine, plus vitamin B complex. People with an irregularity or malfunction of the pituitary gland have been shown to be lacking in these minerals and vitamins. All glands are subservient to the pituitary. It is therefore necessary to check all other glands when any irregularities are noted in the pituitary area of the iris. Any brown or dark deterioration on the iris in the pituitary indicates that both alfalfa, a mild food diet, as well as a cleansing formula are essential in order to make improvement in the condition.

Pathologically related signs: fluid retention, congestion in the head area, congestion in any or all other glands, wavy lines on the iris, atlas and axis vertebrae, breast, cecum, penis, scrotum, and spleen.

The submaxillary glands are either of two glands that secrete saliva, one gland to each side just below the ear, under the jawbone. The one on the left shows on the left iris in zones 3 and 4 between 45° and 55°. The right gland shows on the right iris between 305° and 315°.

Pathologically related signs: arm, axilla, bronchials, ears, hand, jaw, larynx, lens, mastoid, neck, and tonsils.

The thyroid is a large gland in front of and on either side of the trachea. It secretes the hormone thyroxine, and iodine hormone, which regulates the growth and fluids of the body. On the left iris the thyroid shows at 285°, on the right iris at 75°. The herbs used to make changes in the thyroid are kelp or dulse, (a deep sea lettuce). Kelp or dulse are best taken in the liquid form when some people need up to 70 or more tablets, (one drop equals one tablet). Persons with a hyper thyroid, or thin type, need approximately 4 to 6 tablets or drops of kelp or dulse. Persons with a hypothyroid, or fat type, need approximately 20 to 70 or more drops. It requires 20 tablets of kelp or 20 drops of liquid natural iodine to equal 16 mg tablet of thyroxine drug. Thyroxine is a drug that is hard on the heart and should not be used if there is a problem with the heart. Cancer in the gland requires cleansing formulas and a mild food diet as well as iodine.

Pathologically related signs: any or all of the other major glands – primarily the parathyroid's, wavy lines in the iris, fluid retention, toxic bowel, heart, lungs, bronchials, submaxillary glands, ears, atlas and axis vertebrae, jaw, larynx, lens, pharynx, and spleen.

CHAPTER 12

LESIONS

Open lesions indicate inherent weaknesses if they are just a color shade darker than the color of the iris. Any darkening shades down into the lower layers indicate chronic deterioration in varying stages. Open lesions heal faster than closed lesions because the closed lesions indicate a closed area of weakness in the body not as easily accessible to cleansing waste into the blood stream. Sometimes closed lesions will be the last to show healing, even though all other areas of the eye indicates healing is happening. Lesions that are chronic will sometimes knit, having the appearance of a darned sock. Lines will weave closer and closer at times closing the lesion when corrective measures in diet and herbs are taken; other times they may clean to a color shade darker than the eye and remain, because the weakness remains. Chronic deterioration usually begins on the outside edge of the lesion moving from outside to the center in varying stages of chronic color from yellow to brown to black, but as it begins to heal, white will appear on the top and around the edges with the knitting line appearance. Colors underneath gradually lighten and colors on top become whiter until they disappear.

Open lesions are easier to change than closed lesions simply because waste has a way out. The way to remove the waste is to use mild foods and cleansing herbs.

CLOSED LESIONS

A closed lesion is more serious than an open lesion and is more difficult to heal. When white knitting lines begin to appear on a closed lesion it is a good indication that the problem can be solved.

CHAPTER 13

PARASITES

Radii Solaris   *Parasites*

Radii solaris spokes look like a dark, sharply cut line which can be major or minor. These lines or spokes sometimes extend from pupil to peripheral border of the iris, and sometimes they are short lines extending out from the autonomic wreath. Radii solaris lines have been considered to be difficult to overcome mainly because iridologists had not been aware that they were an indication of parasites. Heavy parasite involvement in the particular part of the body where they appear, show up as the radii solaris spokes. When parasites are killed, the lines begin to flatten and have a fuzzy appearance and lighten in color eventually to white, then disappear altogether. The so-called radiation lines which are wider than radii solaris spokes are also involved with parasites.

Parasites were a definite pathological concept in ancient Egyptian medicine as shown by the graphic reproduction of animals in mural paintings, comprising an important part of certain hieroglyphics that indicate disease. Ra, the sun God, fell sick because of a worm born from his sputum. When the parasite is not visible, an invisible worm is imagined.

During the period when Egypt passed under domination of Persia, the decay in medicine began. The conquerors tried to preserve ancient traditions in medicine but the physician was too closely attached to the religious priests and government rule. At this change of hands, the brilliant medical practices decayed into sorcery and charlatan drug vendors, similar to what has happened in the past 50 years to our own society. Our grandmothers were well acquainted with de-worming their children, but today we only de-worm our pets.

Where cancer parasites (Progenitor Cryptocides, etc.) Are present, cancer formulas are used. Additional herbs such as black walnut may also be used. Where salmonella and trichinosis are present, and herbal pumpkin formula may be used. Where lupus, malaria, or leprosy are present, the herb black walnut is the best choice.

Lines will fuzz off then go to white, then disappear as parasites are killed. Pumpkin seed and herbal pumpkin formulas will usually take care of radii solaris spokes, but it takes black walnut to change the radiation lines. The time it takes to rid the body of parasites varies, depending on how deeply entrenched they are. A crisis may occur when mucus sloughs off and may last from two weeks to six or eight months. Sometimes no real crisis is necessary, for the mucus just begins to move a little at a time. As parasites are killed a smelly drainage is caused if parasites are located near a body opening such as in the head area, kidney, vagina, or rectum.

CHAPTER 14

INJURY AND SURGERY

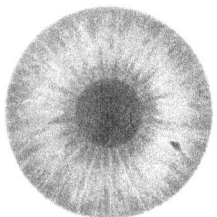

Injury

Injury will show up in many shapes and forms with all lines irregularly crossing natural lines. Toxic waste and deterioration follows the regular line pattern of the iris from pupil to peripheral line but an injury will cross in all or any direction. This is what makes it easily discernible.

For injury-caused scar tissue, vitamin E is used. A person who has been injured must live on a better diet than the average, depending upon where and how much damage was done. Because the body has been altered in some respects in the area of injury, such areas will always be weak and a ready receptacle for the accumulation of toxic waste.

SURGERY

Surgery

A surgery will look at times as though a hole was cut out of the iris of all shapes and sizes. A broken bone will usually show a straight, cut line crossing the bone area where the break occurred. An injury or a surgery may, if permanent damage is done, turn a brown color and remain that way, even though a cleansing diet and herbs are extensively used.

For surgery caused scar tissue vitamin E is used. A person who has had surgery must live on a better diet, depending upon how much surgery has been performed.

CHAPTER 15

DRUGS

Drugs can be easily identified on the iris of the eye by a sodium ring which is a gray-white or brown ring around a peripheral line on the sixth and seventh zones. This ring appears to be superimposed above the top layer. Drugs are also revealed as a red or bright brown circle around the outside edge of the pupil.

What is meant by the word "drug"? In centuries past, the word "drug" was used synonymously with herbs or medicine. As herbs became obsolete to the medical world and were replaced by chemical drugs, herbs were no longer classed as drugs. Some drugs of a chemical nature are made by mixing chemicals with herbs. In this case, the herb is still classed as a drug because of the chemical additive. The chemicals used to make drugs are inorganic substances such as potash, salts, petroleum, and alcohol, as well as drugs made from organic narcotic herbs, such as morphine, caffeine, and nicotine. Some drugs of a narcotic nature are used in the natural state, others are used in conjunction again with chemical salts or potash. In order to identify those botanicals classed as narcotic drugs, we find that all must be given a name ending in "-ine", whether in a natural state or as a mixture with other chemical salts.

Hard narcotic drugs show up on the pupil red ring and whenever brown spots appear to be superimposed over the top layer of the iris. Furthermore, drugs of a narcotic or saline nature both are having an effect on the autonomic wreath when it appears to be chronic in color. Drugs are inhibiting the normal routing of the nerve signals throughout the area of the body where such chronic color appears on the wreath. Sometimes the entire wreath will appear chronic in color: this is another reason for a cleanse to rid the body of the inorganic or drug substances interfering with nerve impulses. Drugs leave a toxic residue in the body or what is called the side effect. When the nervous system is malfunctioning it is with difficulty that the body heals. As drastic changes in the iris occur because of the chemical salts of drugs, the dangers of drugs become more apparent. All of these markings of a brown chronic nature, whether caused by drugs or incorrect eating habits and poor nutrition, are indicative of deteriorating disease. It makes no difference what the cause, for when we see the shadows of doom registering the extent of deterioration in the body, it is time to find out what we have been doing wrong and make a change for the better.

Drugs can be expelled when the body is placed in a fasting or semi-fasting state. As drugs move into circulation, palpitations of the heart will often occur. Care must be taken in the elimination process when many drugs of an extreme toxic or narcotic nature have been taken. Taking care of the heart is important. The use of mild foods and cleansing herbs is a semi-fasting diet.

CHAPTER 16

ACUTE CONDITION

An acute condition in the body is shown on the iris as white over the top of the main color of the iris. A condition such as a cold, flu, measles, mumps, and chickenpox will all register white over most of the iris field. There are varying degrees of white: the more heavily the body is eliminating, the whiter the eyes will become. The iris will register where the body elimination is most actively happening. As the elimination passes out of the body, the white will gradually disappear. Some people have white on their eyes all the time. This type of person has a good ability to eliminate and is in a constant state of elimination. They are always fatigued and weak, the way one feels when he has a cold without the fever. This type of individual could become well rapidly and remain well if he would stop the intake of concentrated or poor foods which the body is always trying to throw off.

When the body is chronically sick and an attempt is made to fast or semi-fast by mild food dieting and herbs, the body will often begin to eliminate, and the eyes will whiten as the elimination begins to take place. "Acute" means toxic waste is on the move in the bloodstream and on its way out. White always means healing, whether nature's forcing an elimination as with a cold to save the life or whether an elimination is caused by a semi-fasting cleanse.

In case of an inflammation, white would show in the inflamed area as white over the top color layer. White appearing deeply between the lines indicates parasites, coupled with an acute pain such as would be caused by lupus, rheumatoid arthritis, or malaria. The white line may turn dark and become a radii solaris, showing only that the parasites are more deeply entrenched and a chronic condition has set in. Because white is always indicative of an acute condition, pain is always involved where white appears. In a case where parasites are involved, the body can remain in an acute, painful condition as the toxic waste just stirs around in the bloodstream and is unable to leave the body. In these cases the parasites must be killed in order to eliminate the waste, because parasites hang onto their food, and most of the waste they live on cannot even be eliminated by fasting. As healing begins to occur, white lines appear where chronic disease is involved. Sometimes healing looks like someone placed a white screen across a brown spot, leaving the brown showing underneath.

In acute inflammation or acute illness, white shows over the original color of the iris. This showing of white means that waste is on the move in the bloodstream. Help nature get the waste out of the body by the use of a fruit only diet, cleansing herbs, and high doses of vitamin C, 1,000 to 2,000 mg an hour. It is also helpful to take a strong laxative and an enema each day until the acute condition is overcome.

Pathologically related signs: pain, fever, and cough.

CHAPTER 17

LIVER, GALLBLADDER

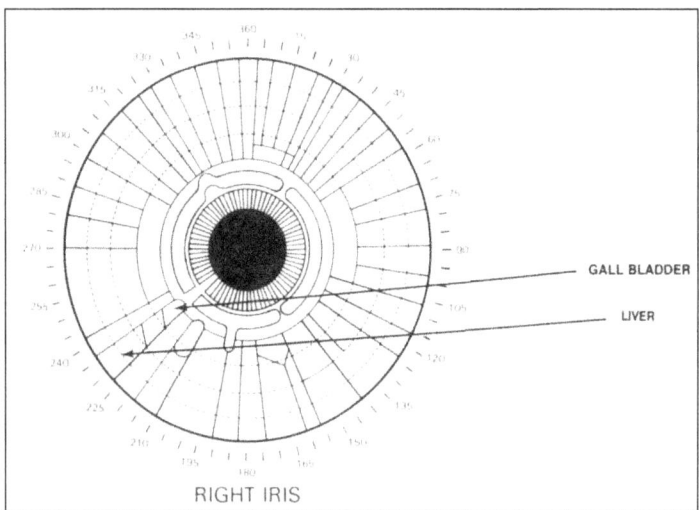

RIGHT IRIS

Any chronic deterioration showing on the liver and gallbladder causes a difficulty with healing. Sometimes the bowel is blocked, causing the liver to malfunction. The bowel area must be checked to see if it shows a toxic condition. If so this would be the first thing to clear out for the liver to empty and clean. When chronic color shows in the gallbladder, gallstones are expected to be the problem.

The liver is the largest glandular organ of the body. It is located just below the two lungs, almost directly below the heart, and just in front of the stomach. The liver is important because it secretes bile and has an important function in fat and carbohydrate metabolism it also contains a substance essential to the production of red blood cells the liver is located between 227° to 235° in zone 5 on the right iris.

To heal the liver and gallbladder it is important to use a mild food diet and a cleansing herbal formula. Gallbladder purge may also be needed. The gallbladder purge is used to empty the gallbladder of stones so that normal elimination can be carried on. The other place to look in conjunction with liver and gallbladder would be the duodenum. If there is an ulceration showing or a chronic color, slippery elm is the herb that is soothing to an ulceration. Goldenseal, saffron, lemons, and raw beet juice all activate and clean the liver. The minerals that have been used to help heal the liver are sodium, fluorine, potassium, and magnesium.

Pathologically related signs: colon, eyes, ears, appendix, stomach, gallbladder, heart, skin, axilla, back, bile duct, diaphragm, esophagus, peritoneum, ribs, albumin, and abdominal wall.

The gallbladder is the organ that is attached to the liver in which excess bile is concentrated for the digestion of fat. The gallbladder is located on the right iris at about 230° in zone 3.

Pathologically related signs: liver, colon, eyes, ears, appendix, stomach, heart, skin, bile duct, diaphragm, and esophagus.

CHAPTER 18

KIDNEYS

When the kidney area appears white, and inflammation is in progress. White on any given area indicates acute and is always associated with pain. When inflammation appears to be a gray, metallic color it indicates an over-acidic condition. Any deterioration showing from yellow to black in color indicates kidneys are in trouble. The shadow or just a shade darker than the eye color showing either in a lesion or in the lines from the color to the periphery in the kidney area means that the person will always have to take special care of his weak kidneys. This type of person often wets the bed as a child until far past the acceptable age.

The kidney is a glandular organ in which there are a pair. The function of the kidney is to separate waste and water products from the blood. This waste and water is then secreted as urine. The kidney is located in the body in the upper abdominal cavity, one on either side of the abdominal cavity. The left kidney shows on the left iris between 184° and 196° in zone 4. The right kidney shows on the right iris between 162° and 174° in zone 4.

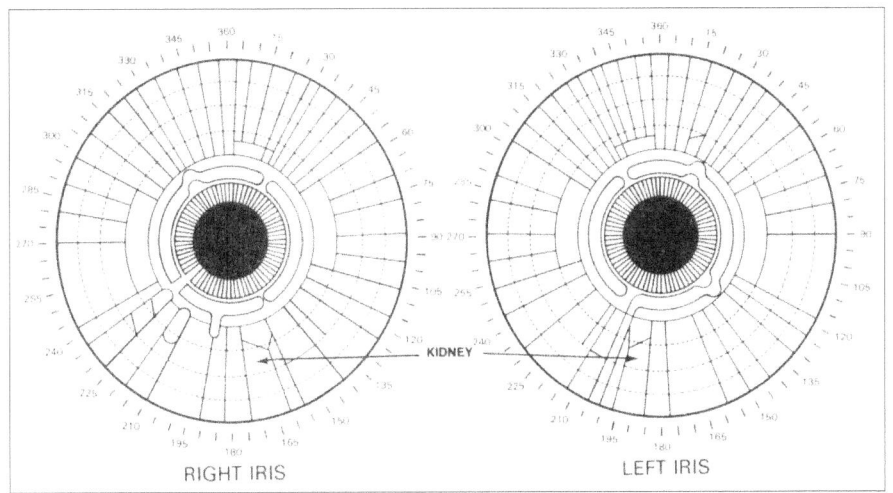

RIGHT IRIS

LEFT IRIS

KIDNEY

When there is infection in the kidneys, the same procedure should be followed as with any acute inflammation: to help nature remove the waste from the body fruit only, cleansing herbs, high doses of vitamin C and enemas. When there is deterioration, cleansing herb formulas and mild food along with uric acid removing herbs such as saffron and dandelion may be used.

If the problem is determined to be kidney stones, a purge of the kidneys may be used. This is accomplished by discontinuing all eating, except lemon juice in a small amount of water, continued until the stone or stones are dissolved. It is not usually necessary to take lemon juice longer than 12 to 14 hours. The lemon juice will act on the kidney stones as water acts on rock salt, melting away the sharp edges. The sharp edges of a kidney stone cut like glass on their way through the urethra on their way to the bladder, causing swelling and intense pain. With a kidney stone, the pain can be as severe as a difficult delivery of a baby. A man who has passed a kidney stone knows what a difficult birth can be like. The taking of lemon juice is such an easy thing and works so well, it is hard for me to understand why medical science has not discovered so simple a remedy. For ongoing weakness and infection in the kidneys, juniper is the herb of choice.

Pathologically related signs: albumin, abdominal wall, adrenals, submaxillary glands, back, bladder, eyes, hip, parathyroid, penis, peritoneum, prostate, ribs, urethra, and uric acid.

CHAPTER 19

BONES

On the iris chart, the bony areas are well-defined: shoulder, scapula, thoracic (rib cage), spinal, leg (thigh, knee, and foot), hand and arm, pelvis, and the neck are represented (the latter on the medulla). The top of the head appears at 360°, back of the head towards 30°, jaw, nose, face, and skin area close to the periphery. A break will cross the normal lines of the iris and can show if the bone has been shattered or broken clean. When deterioration has set in, the break will appear brown or black. Otherwise, crisscross, jagged, odd shaped markings will appear, depending upon what kind of a break.

Often an old break, even one that was well set, will be susceptible to arthritis and will also appear to be brown in color. If it is damaged, deterioration of bone and surrounding tissue, the brown color may never change. If it is an arthritic condition, irreversible changes may occur in the bone shape. But the brown showing deterioration may leave the iris. The brown or black, if there is arthritis in the bone, will show on the sixth zone of the bone area.

Hypercalcemia will appear gray-white in color. If it is general throughout the whole body, the entire iris color will appear to be gray-white on the top of the color of the eye. When it is specifically causing site problems, a gray glandular appearance will appear on either side of the pupil. A calcium problem in the body, whether it is settling in the arteries, in the joints, or in the tissues, involves the adrenal and parathyroid glands.

In order to regulate the correct calcium metabolism, glands need to be properly functioning and secreting necessary hormones. In order to bring calcium back to normal ossification when the body is not producing adequate hormones, herbal hormone-type herbs will sustain life the way insulin does in a diabetic. For extreme uric acid and lactic acid buildup, saffron and dandelion are helpful herbs. The adrenal hormone-type herb is licorice, while the parathyroid hormone-type herbs are alfalfa and kelp.

Osteoporosis is a calcium lack where insufficient calcium causes the body to begin (activated by the parathyroid glands) to leach calcium from the bones in order to maintain correct calcium levels in the blood. The bones then become hollow and brittle. This often happens with old people who live on bland diets not rich in calcium and other minerals. This is a cause of much of the senility in old age. For the brain to function well, blood calcium must be kept at correct levels even in a hypercalcemia condition where calcium is deposited in the body, the person could have too low a level of calcium in the blood. This is the cause of the mental breakdown common to the hypo and hyperglycemia type.

An arc or crescent appearing across the upper portion of the iris brain area – looking as if the white pulled down over the upper iris obscuring the peripheral line – indicates that senility is beginning due to the lack of calcium and oxygen to the brain. By helping the glands and calcium metabolism in the body, senility can often be thwarted. Niacin also helps to give circulation to the brain area. Exercise on a slant board, inversion bed, or yoga headstand, with correct breathing, is also helpful to bring more oxygen to the brain. Sometimes, however, the arc is caused by brain damage, and senility is the result. An osteoporosis, or the hollowing out of the bone, appears on the body structures of the body of the iris as a pit-like appearance, like cement that has not been troweled enough. The addition of calcium and related minerals, which cause calcium to be utilized in the body, will readily improve this condition.

CHAPTER 20

ANEMIA

The arc that designates anemia is often accompanied by a scurf rim. The combination of the two, places an added burden on the internal skin and other organs of elimination. This should indicate that toxic waste is accumulating in the area of the arc and has had difficulty in moving out. Anemia means an encumbrance of toxic waste in the blood. It is interesting to note that when the white blood count is high and the system is cleansed with herbs and mild food, the white count goes down and the red count goes up. When the system is cleaned, the arc clears off of the iris. According to the writings of most iridologists, anemia is considered to be associated with arcus senilis. The arcus senilis may appear anywhere on the iris for example, it would look like an arc created by the sclera or white of the eye being pulled down over the iris in a crescent that obscures the peripheral line.

If a person is anemic, the iris of the eye will remain white most of the time, with the exception of when a person is on a continual cleanse. Continual mucus waste in the blood can lead to leukemia. To change such a condition, the intake of mucus forming food must be stopped and treated the same as a cold until the iris changes to its normal color.

The term anemia is not correctly understood. Unless there has been hemorrhaging, the need for iron is very small. This is the same reason women who menstruate need more iron than men. The term "brain anemia" has been used among iridologists to denote the arc as in arcus senilis, and if the arc appears any other place obscuring the periphery or part of the circumference, it is called anemia. My view differs in that I call it simply a lack of circulation to the area where the arc may appear. Improvement of circulation will change the arc in all areas, except in the brain area where there has been brain damage. Even then it can be possible if all situations are correct and a continuing effort is made. There are people who eventually regain normal functions after a stroke with little or no permanent damage.

Medical science looks at the white blood count, and if it is high, they believe iron is needed so they prescribe iron from an inorganic or a non-chelated source. The body immediately attempts to rid itself of the toxic poison. The white corpuscle's (acting as a holding system for toxic waste) move much of the waste already in the blood (causing the white appearance on the iris) back into the bodies lymphatic system, in order to eradicate the poison. The person feels stronger, not because of the iron, but because the waste which was on its way out of the body causing the weakness of acute sickness, is suddenly and quickly moved out of the blood. When another blood test is taken the white count will have gone down and the red count gone up. The same thing can be done with a sunlamp or a sun bath, but rather than pushing the waste back into the lymph, the toxic waste is removed by the sunlamp or sunrays and the white count goes down. As the body detoxifies on a cleansing program, the iris will whiten on top of the normal color until waste is removed from the body. The iris will then change to normal color.

Sometimes in the process of detoxifying, the iris will whiten to anemia, pernicious anemia, and leukemia color white. If a blood test were taken at this time, the doctor would say the person had any of the three, depending upon the extent of toxic elimination. If detoxification cleansing is continued, the blood cleans and the white disappears from the iris. The tongue will whiten in the same way and as the body cleans, the coating on the tongue disappears also. The iris and tongue can be closely monitored while on a cleansing program and therefore be better controlled. Too much waste in the bloodstream can kill, therefore close monitoring can tell a person when to slow down the elimination and when to increase it. More fruits increase elimination while more vegetables slow down the process somewhat.

CHAPTER 21

SCURF RIM

The scurf rim suggests the condition of the skin. Anytime the peripheral line is wider than a pencil line this is called a scurf rim, and it may widen as far as the fifth zone. The uniformity of depths can vary all around the circumference of the iris, indicating that the skin may be better in one place than another. The darker and more defined the color and the wider the ring, the greater the impairment of skin function and the retention of toxic waste just under the skin. If the color is only a shade darker than the color of the iris and a scurf rim is showing to any extent, this is only inherent weakness. Other problems will result if the bowel and kidneys cannot carry off the waste properly. The skin is the third kidney, and when it is not functioning well, the entire body suffers. Wherever there is an incursion of the scurf rim, the area of incursion becomes more readily toxic in that part of the body. When rosary nodules appear to have split over into the scurf rim showing a white line, this indicates swelling or fluid buildup in the tissues of that area of the body, revealing these white lines on the iris.

When the scurf rim shows only a darker color than the color of the eye, this is weakness. It will result in an added burden on the internal skin as well as bowel and kidney. Stimulation of the skin, steam or sweat baths, sun baths, massage, or a bath and a good towel rub will help solve the scurf rim problem. When the problem is chronic, mild food and cleansing herbs should be used, along with those things listed above.

CHAPTER 22

LYMPHATIC ROSARY

The lymphatic rosary on the iris appears like globs or nodules of white, yellow, or brown beads strung around the sixth zone. Sometimes they connect all the way around, other times they are disconnected and show only sparsely around the circumference on the sixth zone. Anytime these globs show on the iris anywhere on this zone, it is an indication of an accumulation of mucus waste in the lymph of the body. If the color is extremely white – almost blue – and appears to be superimposed on the top of the fibers of the iris, it is considered as an index of arsenic retention in the lymph system. When the lymphatic rosary appears white, yellow or brown and has a thickening of the fibers themselves, this indicates lymph congestion. Often there is arsenic retention as well as mucus congestion of the lymph, making it difficult to distinguish. The arsenic retained in the lymph is related to neuritis conditions and will become neuritis later as it becomes more chronic. It can also be related to arthritis.

There are seven zones from pupil to peripheral line. The sixth zone, where the lymphatic rosary is found, has to do with circulation. When circulation is poor, the lymph nodes and the body begin to retain waste. As waste is retained in the lymph, the thyroid works overtime to send iodine into the body to kill germs living in accumulating mucus waste. When thyroid activity is increased, pituitary activity is decreased, as if it were on a balance scale: overactivity of the thyroid increases oxidation to assist the body in expelling waste, much the same way we breathe faster when we have a cold or fever. When the thyroid gland is overactive, the pituitary decreases its activity causing a slow-down of all other glandular activity. All glands are subservient to the pituitary, and an all-out effort is directed through the thyroid to fight against bacteria in lymphatic waste which is accumulating, as indicated by the presence of a lymphatic rosary. The spleen is also noted in conjunction with the lymphatic rosary. The spleen is the organ of the body related to the production of red blood cells, but another activity of the spleen is to retain waste from the lymphatic system. It is much like a holding tank. When the lymphatic waste becomes alarmingly full, the spleen acts like a vacuum, drawing as much waste as possible to itself until such time as the body can overcome the waste. At that time the spleen will then eliminate retained waste. The appendix does a similar thing with the colon when an impaction in the ascending colon threatens to cause a backup of waste into the small intestines.

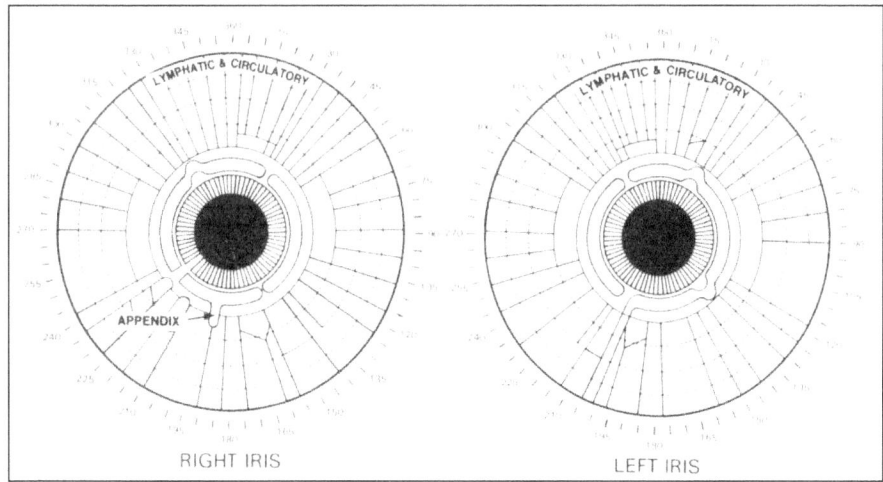

The appendix protects the body as an overflow valve, because when waste backs up into the small intestines where absorption of nutrients takes place, it could poison the whole body. When the spleen and lymphatic system become full, the body immune system is lowered. When the spleen area in the lymphatic rosary on the iris appears full all the way around and an overlay of white is superficially imposed on the top of the color of the iris, this is indicative of Hodgkin's disease.

A problem in the lymph system can develop into Hodgkins disease, even if the rosary remains white for too long. To clean the entire lymphatic system a mild food diet and cleansing herbs, particularly laxatives are used. Flush the body lymph. When chronic cholesterol is the cause, lecithin helps to emulsify and loosen fatty wastes in the arteries. Check for lymphatic rosary across bony structures indicating arthritis. Check glands areas for incorrect calcium balance. Any imbalance can cause further calcium buildup and hardening arteries.

CHAPTER 23

ALPHABETICAL LISTING
OF BODY PARTS

ABDOMINAL WALL

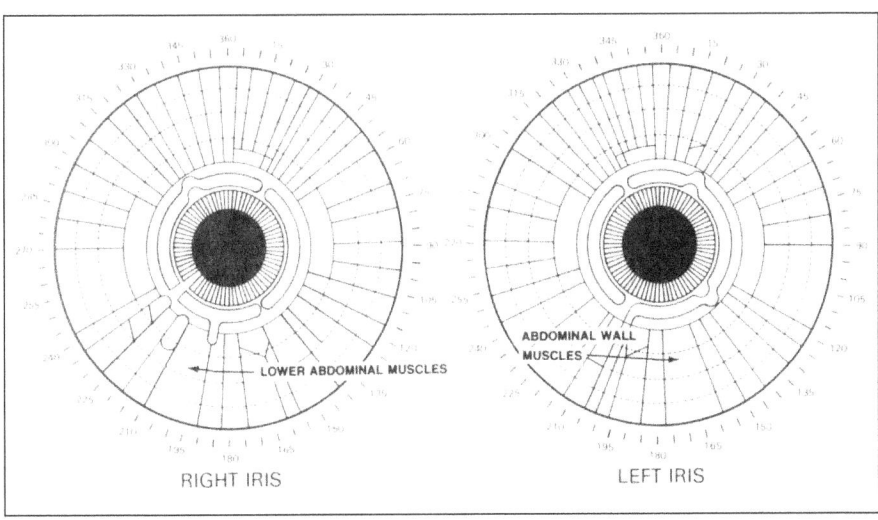

The abdominal area is often the area to register surgical markings because so much surgery is performed on that area of the body. Markings other than nerve rings which cross the lines that extend from pupil to peripheral indicate surgery or injury. Sometimes the iris will look like there is a whole in the area where surgery has been performed. Sometimes only a line appears, depending upon whether or not an organ has been removed. If there has been permanent damage to the area of injury or surgery, the area will darken and remain so, no matter what the person does to try to change such markings. The injured or surgically treated area will go white immediately upon injury or surgery, and then if tissue has been damaged permanently, it will darken to a depth of color brown to black, depending upon the extent of damage. Color in a lesion which has darkened into the lower layers denotes deterioration in the bodily area of the lesion.

On the right iris the abdominal muscles are located between 190° and 210°. On the left iris the abdominal muscles are located between 170° and 175°.

A mild food diet may be used when other areas are involved relating to the abdominal wall. Vitamin E taken internally helps to overcome scar tissue, and used externally will help the scar disappear.

Pathologically related signs: note the color of the small intestinal area, pancreas, liver, stomach, male and female organs, check for head congestion, headaches, kidneys, and adrenal glands.

ALBUMIN

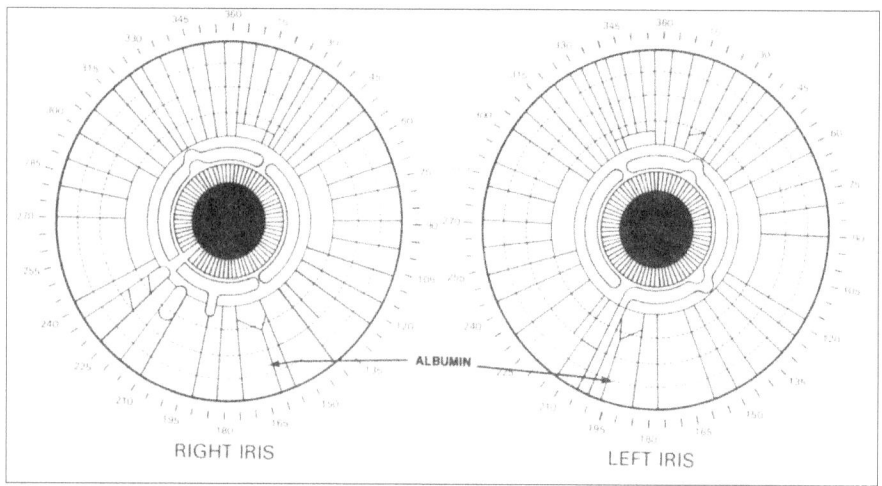

RIGHT IRIS   LEFT IRIS

Albuminuria

Albumin in the urine is considered by medical standards to be a useful substance and consider that some people have albumin in their urine naturally without evidence of kidney disease. They even note that infections and violent exercise can cause albumin in the urine. Medical science even understands that if there is too much albumin this suggests that the kidney filtering apparatus is defective, yet they still persist in the age old idea that it is somehow useful and must be replaced by a protein diet when it is spilled off.

Professor Arnold Ehret said that such a theory borders on insanity. The protein theory is becoming obsolete. It will not be long until science realizes that albumin is a waste mucus product, and that is why the flow of albumin is heaviest after exercise or infectious disease. Albumin is present when the iris appears white in the area of the kidney section where it is designated on the chart.

Changes in albuminuria can often take place simply by drinking a glass of warm distilled water with lemon juice. If a more serious elimination is going on, it may be treated as a cold.

Albumin is the toxic mucus waste of the body: any number of complex proteins found in muscle, milk, eggs, and in many vegetable fluids and tissue. They are coagulated by heat, consist of carbon, nitrogen, oxygen, sulfur, and hydrogen. They dissolve in water.

Pathologically related signs: kidneys, bladder, liver, heart, bowel, back pain, and descending colon.

ARM

Deterioration, such as cancer or arthritis, will show in the arm area of the iris as brown or black. When there is any infection in the arm, the iris will whiten in the designated arm area. Often when there is a condition of swollen glands or congestion of a head cold, the arm area will also white. The kidneys may also be noted in such cases for whiteness as the body tries to eradicate the mucus waste of a cold, for the kidneys and bladder are much overworked.

The arm is one of two upper limbs of the body, the part between the shoulder and hand. The left-hand is represented in the left iris, the right hand in the right iris. The left-hand shows in zone 3 at 118° to 125°. The right-hand shows in zone 3 at 235° to 242°.

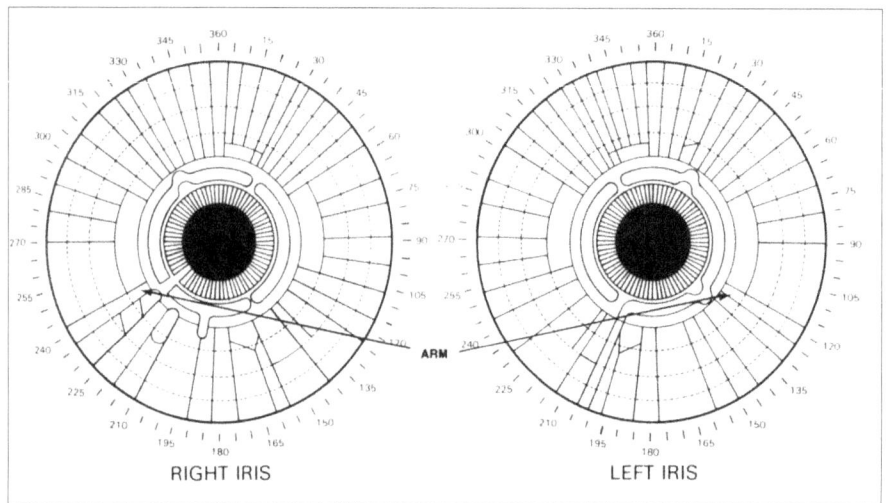

RIGHT IRIS   LEFT IRIS

A mild food diet may be used along with cleansing herbs for chronic problems. Treat as with a cold for acute problems.

Pathologically related signs: submaxillary gland, kidney, bladder, bowel, atlas and axis vertebrae, throat, head, heart, hand, and wrist.

ATLAS AND AXIS VERTEBRAE

These two main vertebrae in the neck which support the weight of the head can cause many problems when they are out of alignment. Some chronic diseases are a direct result of the injury and inherent organic fault in these areas.

The Atlas vertebrae is the first cervical vertebrae, the vertebrae that supports the head. The atlas vertebrae is located in zone 3 between 20° and 25° on the left iris, and 335° to 343° on the right iris. A good chiropractor or acupressurist is most helpful.

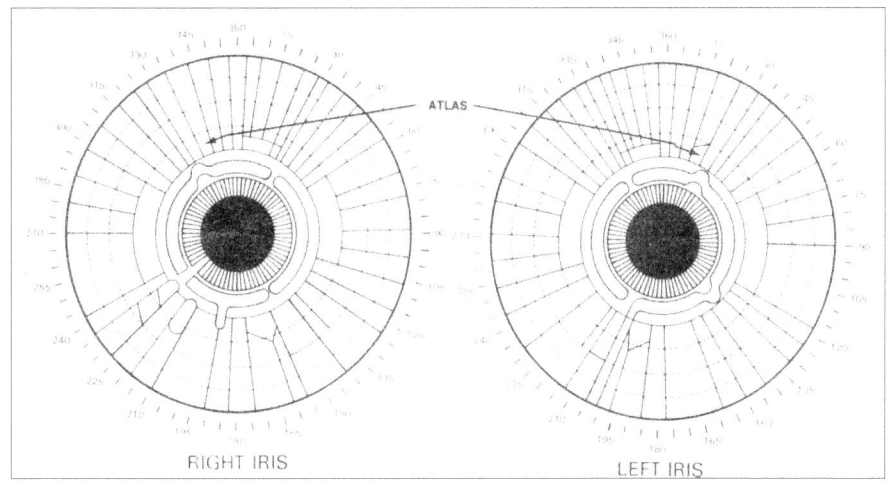

RIGHT IRIS

LEFT IRIS

Pathologically related signs: eyes, ears, head congestion, throat, thyroid, parathyroid, pituitary, submaxillary gland, back, legs, neck, and nose.

AXILLA

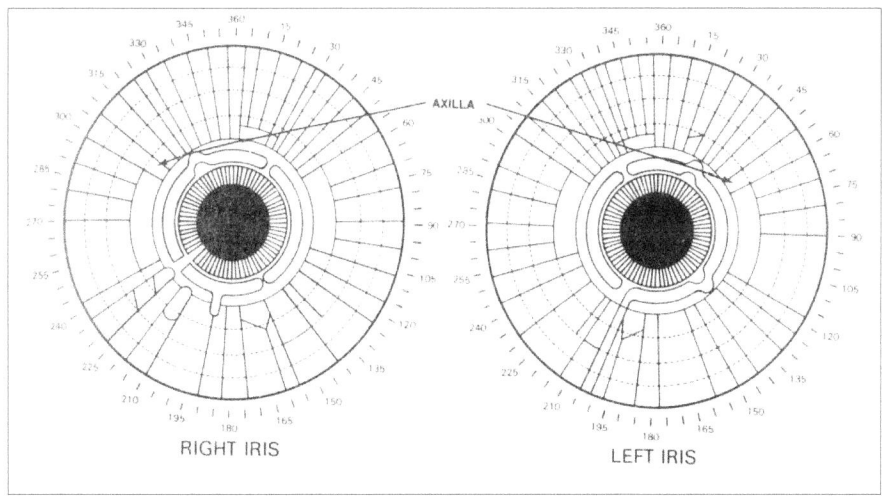

RIGHT IRIS

LEFT IRIS

The most commonly associated phenomenon noted in relation to the axilla is underarm perspiration. The armpit is one of the main areas of perspiration of the body. While the body is cleansing, or if the body is filthy, the armpit can be most offensive, so man has devised a way to shut off perspiration with deodorants. Congestion in the head, chest, and heart areas could be directly related to the use of deodorants which inhibit the body's ability to throw off waste through the underarm.

The axillary artery is located in a space pyramidal between the upper side part of the chest and the axis plane of the arm. "Axilla" means pertaining to the armpit. On the left iris it is located in zone 3 between 55° and 63°, on the right iris between 105° and 140°.

Washing everyday helps to overcome offensive odor. Exercise and an occasional steam or sauna bath helps the body eliminate through the axilla (under arm).

Pathologically related signs: head congestion, back, liver, heart, lungs, submaxillary glands, mastoid, ears, and eyes.

BACK

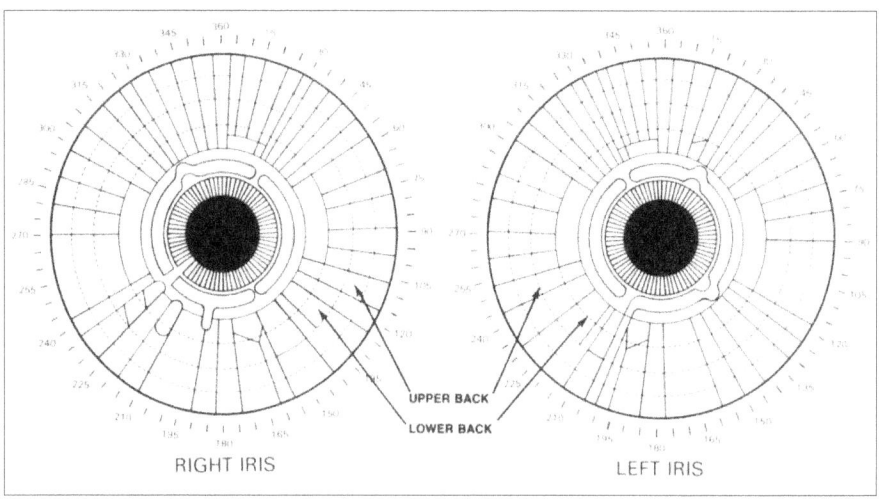

RIGHT IRIS

UPPER BACK
LOWER BACK

LEFT IRIS

The back shows up on the iris of the eye in zones 3, 4, and 5. The top of the spine starts in zone 3 and ends in zone 5, on the left iris. On the right iris the top of the spine starts at zone 3 and ends in zone 5 also. On the left iris between 220° and 255°. On the right iris between 105° and 140°.

Exercise is of the utmost importance. A good chiropractor, touch therapy, inversion therapy and a cleansing diet should help. With lower back pain colonic irrigation and cleansing herbs and psyllium are used.

Upper Back

Much upper back pain is related to neck problems and can also be associated with the heart. When nerve rings cross the spinal areas, a person can almost tell his chiropractor where to adjust.

Middle Back

Pain in the middle back is associated with scoliosis, liver, kidneys, and adrenals, and pancreas.

Lower Back

Pain in the lower back is almost always associated with impaction in the bowel, male and female problems, or bladder problems. When people clean out their colons, lower back pain generally leaves. Even when the back seems to be thrown out by sciatic pain it can be traced to bowel impactions.

Pathologically related signs: axis and atlas vertebrae, spinal nerve impingement, scoliosis, liver, kidneys, headache pain, adrenals, bladder infections, male and female problems, bowel impactions, axilla, and knee.

BILE DUCT

Bile causes efficient absorption of fats and also alkalizes the intestines. Bile does not drip steadily. Nature uses muscular valves to control the flow of bile. The gallbladder acts like a holding area until sight, taste, and good smell cause the gallbladder to empty.

Because of an incorrect diet of too much oil and starch, the gallbladder fluids may crystallize, forming gallstones. If large stones try to move through the bile duct, it may rupture.

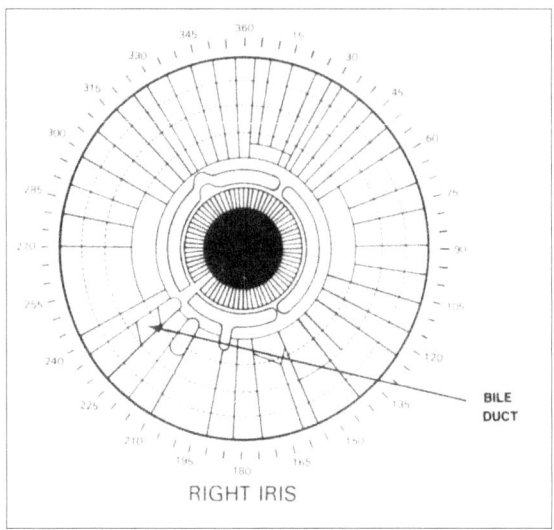

BILE DUCT

RIGHT IRIS

The bile duct shows on the right iris mostly in zone 4 at 227° to 235°. The bile duct is that part of the body which transports bile secreted in the liver and concentrated in the gallbladder to the small intestine. Bile assists the digestions of fats by emulsifying fatty materials. (See Liver and Gallbladder.)

Pathologically related signs: gallbladder, liver, adrenals, and stomach.

BLADDER

The bladder is subject to infection because waste from the body is continually passing through in the form of urine. Women often have bladder infections because of poor sanitary habits, and sometimes bladder infections are caused by impactions in the lower bowel causing absorption of toxic matter through the intestinal wall into the bladder. The bladder may be injured during a difficult childbirth, or it may be subject to tumors, stones, or congenital malformations. It is noted by any darkening of the bladder area of the iris. Urine becomes cloudy or bloody when there is infection in the bladder. Pain always accompanies infection with frequency of urination and a burning pain.

The iris will appear white over the bladder area when infection is present.

The urinary bladder is a sac made up of muscle-membrane. This sac acts as a reservoir for the urine. Its size varies according to the amount of liquid it contains. On the left iris it is located between 213° and 218° in zones 3 and 4. On the right iris it is located between 135° and 142° in zones 3 and 4.

Goldenseal root is used to stop bleeding bladders, as it has an antibiotic effect on infection. Use approximately 2 to 4 capsules every four hours. It is not a good idea to use cayenne for bladder infection. Slippery Elm works very well to soothe and overcome pain. An enema will usually help as much as anything to overcome the infection. (See kidneys.)

Pathologically related signs: kidneys, back pain, female or male genital organs, vagina, urethra, lower bowel, albumin, submaxillary glands, breast, hip, and peritoneum.

BREAST

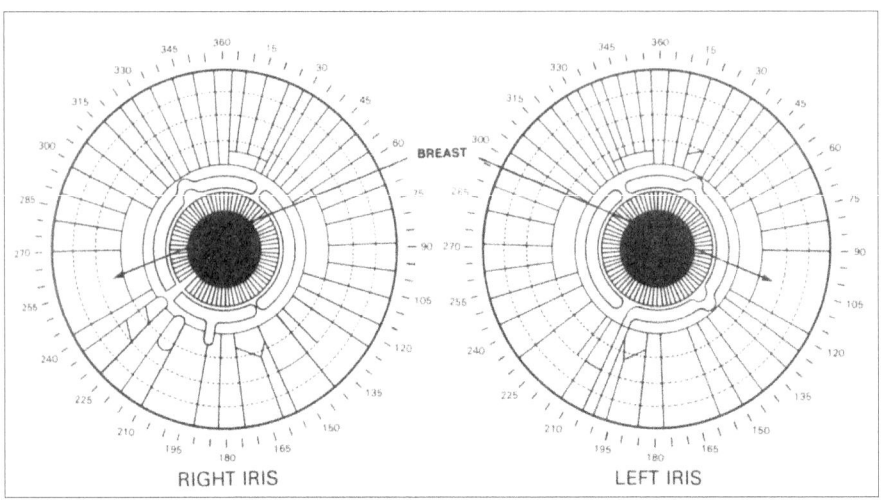

RIGHT IRIS   LEFT IRIS

1 million or more women in the United States have had a mastectomy of one or both breasts. Cancer of the breast strikes 1 in 18 women; therefore, close attention should be paid to the breast area of the iris. Deterioration can be noted on the iris long before symptoms develop. In most cases when cancer has reached the symptom level it is already too late. As a woman is going through a cleanse on mild food and cleansing herbs, if she has had any problems in the breast, the breast will be the last to cleanse. With iridology the problem can be closely monitored, thereby allaying discouragement.

On a female, the breast is either of two milk-secreting glands protruding from the upper front part of her body. A male has corresponding glands, but his are undeveloped. On the iris they show at about 105° on the left iris, on the right iris at about 255°, in zones 4 and 5 on both.

Pathologically related signs: female organs, adrenals, pituitary gland, parathyroid's, bowel, bladder, lungs, ribs, sternum.

BRONCHIALS

The lungs and bronchials can become infected with parasites. Hydatid disease, a disease of variety of tapeworm, invades the lungs and is contracted by handling animals. Hookworm, on the other hand, begins in the lining of the small intestines and spreads throughout the body and is often the cause of chronic bronchitis.

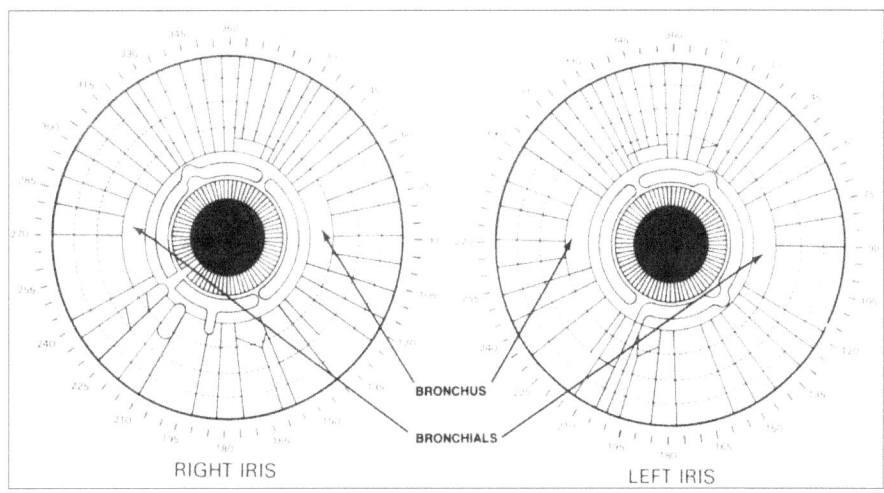

BRONCHUS

BRONCHIALS

RIGHT IRIS

LEFT IRIS

Bronchitis, like asthma, may be caused by inhaling certain irritants such as smog, smoke, or chemicals. Some plants and pollens act like an irritant and produce a forced cleanse in certain people. It is never been my belief that allergies were the cause of problems; rather, that the person's body is full of toxic waste and the flower pollen or whatever merely triggers an elimination. Many people who have had allergies for years do not ever have them again once they have cleaned their bodies with herbs and mild food. When bronchitis continues over long periods of time, pus can become hardened and obstruct the bronchials and the eventual result will be emphysema.

The bronchials are either of two main branches of the windpipe – the right one is shorter than the left. They carry air from the mouth and nose to the lungs. On the iris of both eyes they show at between 58° and 106° and 224° and 397°.

A parasite formula or herbal pumpkin or garlic, along with a mild food diet and cleansing herbs, may be used to help with problems in the bronchials. High doses of vitamins, along with colon therapy, also have been known to be effective.

Pathologically related signs: Larynx, trachea, lungs, pleura, submaxillary glands, mastoid, eyes, nose, ears, colon, and esophagus.

CLAVICLE

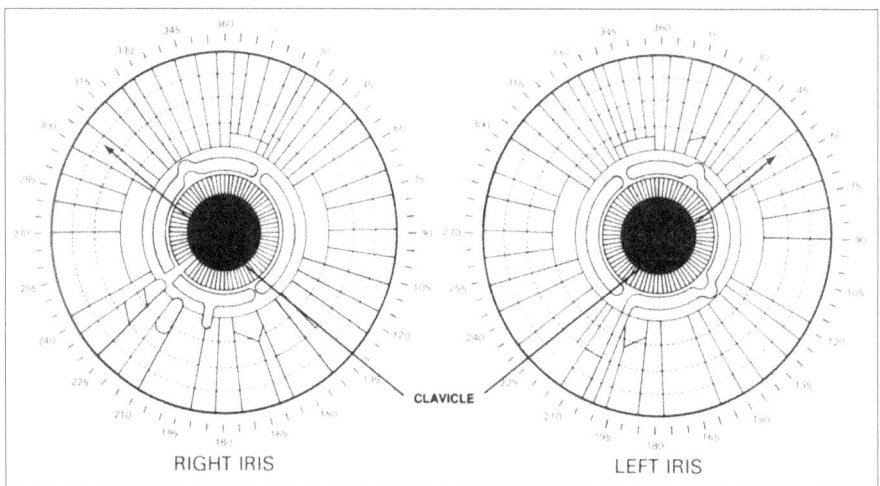

RIGHT IRIS   LEFT IRIS

The clavicle is a small bone connecting the shoulder blade with the breastbone. It is more commonly called the collarbone. The left iris corresponding with the left side of the body shows the left clavicle at 55° to 63° in zone 4. The right iris corresponding with the right side of the body shows the right clavicle in about zone 3 at 297° 305°.

DIAPHRAGM

The diaphragm is that portion of the tendons and muscles that separates the thorax from the lower abdomen. On the left iris it is located at 95° to 105° in zones 3, 4, and 5. The right iris at 250° to 260° also in zones 3, 4, and 5.

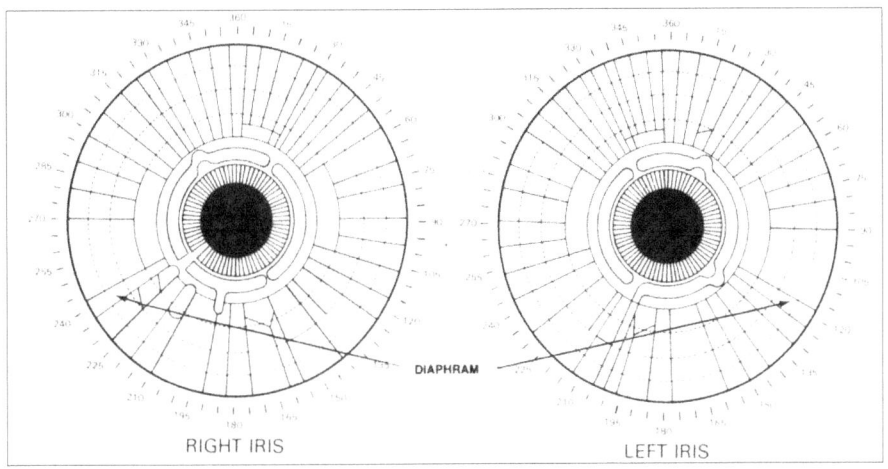

RIGHT IRIS   DIAPHRAM   LEFT IRIS

Everyone has had hiccups. The cause of hiccups are spasms of the diaphragm, resulting from some irritation to the nerves that control the diaphragm. This results in a sharp intake of air which makes the noise that is associated with hiccups. Almost everyone has a cure. Some say to hold your breath as long as possible, others say to take consecutive drinks of water without breathing, still others say to breathe into a paper bag. The principle of these remedies is basically the same, that is to decrease the oxygen and increase the carbon dioxide level in the blood. This should relieve the spastic diaphragm.

A hiatus hernia is a protrusion of part of the stomach through the diaphragm into or next to the esophagus. There are not usually severe symptoms, but there may be a burning sensation, regurgitation of liquid and food, and pain under the breastbone. These symptoms seem to be worse after meals, bending at the waist, or straining the upper body. Also chronic esophagitis, because of regurgitation of acid gastric juices, is associated with hiatus hernia.

The best treatment for hiatal hernia is a mild food diet and manipulation therapy. Another good therapy is to elevate the head of the bed 4 to 6 inches while sleeping. It may be necessary to surgically have the hiatal ring tightened. This is done through the thorax or abdomen. Overeating at night is one of the major causes of hiatus hernia.

Pathologically related signs:* stomach, liver, gallbladder, transverse colon, and shoulder.

EARS

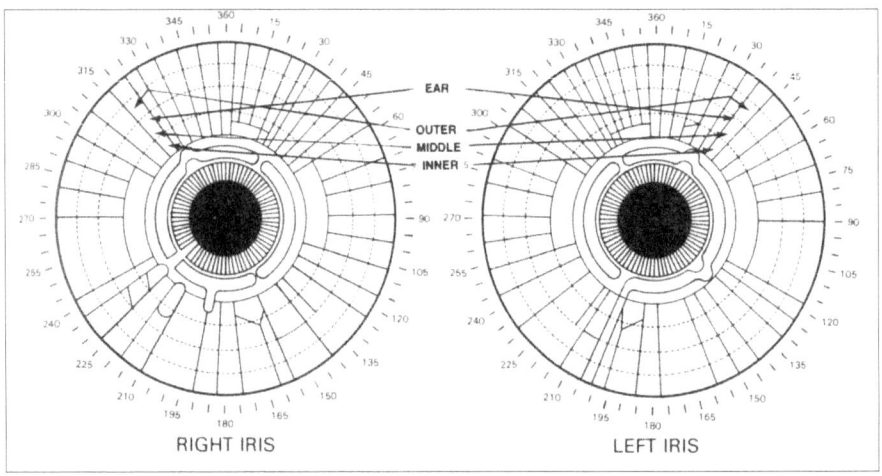

RIGHT IRIS   LEFT IRIS

Problems in the ears and eyes are indicated in a similar manner. However, parasites may have invaded the glands around the ear and neck to the extent that a radiation line will cause eventual prostration of the nerves and can cause nerve deafness. Watch for radii solaris lines and radiation lines on the eye area also.

The ear is that organ of the body that perceives sound. The parts of the ear are: the external ear or the part that can be seen; the auditory canal, the inner ear containing the cochlea and semicircular canals; the middle ear, a cavity connected to the external ear by the tympanic membrane, to the pharynx by the eustachian tube, and to the inner ear by a series of three small bones called the hammer, anvil, and stirrup. The left ear is represented on the iris of the left eye between 315° and 320° in zone 4. The right ear is located between 40° and 45° on the right iris in zone 4.

White on top of the eye color in the area of the ear would mean infection or inflammation. When it is an earache, an ice bag is used to scatter infection away from the ear area. Enemas, fruit diet and laxative herbs will draw the mucus out of the body. If it is a fungus, mullein herb in a tincture or pumpkin seed oil, or black Walnut can be used. Often where there is chronic deterioration showing, a parasite or radiation line will also show. Before the mucus can be moved out, the parasites must first be killed.

Pathologically related signs: liver, gallbladder, submaxillary glands, colon, arteries, throat, nose, eyes, eustachian tubes, atlas and axis vertebrae, axilla, bronchials, cecum, mastoid, mouth, thyroid, tonsils, jaw, and lens.

EYES

The eye section of the iris would show no markings unless there were inherent weakness shadow lines or lesions. When a dark discoloration begins to appear, deterioration of eyesight is beginning to occur. Related organs that can cause site problems need to be checked: kidneys, glands, bowels, and nerve wreath. In order to help sight, all related organs must be helped also. An infection in the eyes or hay fever will appear as a white line on top of the top color layers.

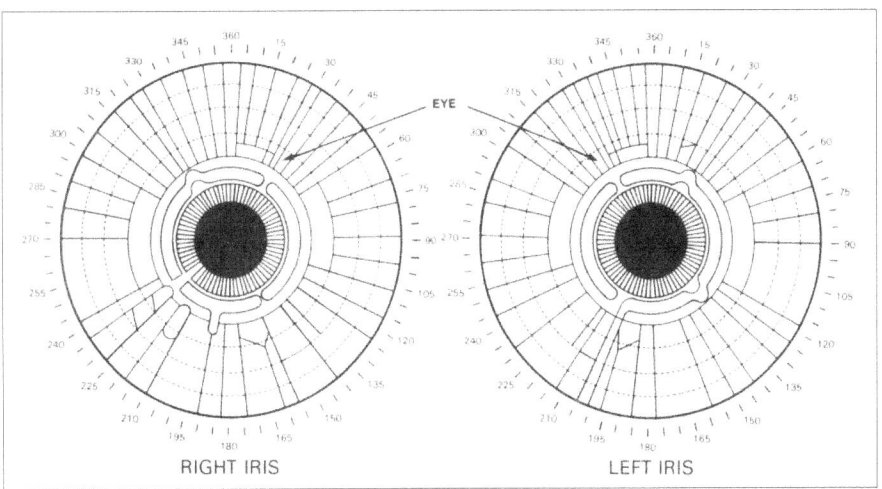

RIGHT IRIS   LEFT IRIS

The eye is the organ of sight. The parts of the eye are, from front to back: cornea, iris, pupil, lens, lens muscle, retina, and optic nerve. The eyes shows in zone 3 between 315° and 323° on the left iris, between 32° and 40° on the right iris.

White showing on the eye area would be inflammation. In order to move inflammation an all fruit diet, herb laxative, enemas, and high vitamin C should be used. Where deterioration is showing, a mild food diet, cleansing herbs formula, vitamin B1, B2, and A are used. Parsley is one of the richest natural sources of vitamin A, even higher than carrots.

Pathologically related signs: brain, ears, nose, throat, liver, gallbladder, kidneys, heart, stomach, colon, eustachian tubes, glands, atlas and axis vertebrae, axilla, bronchials, cecum, lens, mastoid, mouth, pancreas, temple/forehead, and tonsils.

FOOT

Note bony structures of the iris for discoloration, density, arthritis, and damage due to injury or surgery. There are a number of problems associated with the feet from gout, athletes foot, arthritis, to plantar warts. All warts are a result of vitamin A deficiency.

The foot is the end part of the leg on which a person stands and moves. On the left iris the foot is in zone 5 between 175° and 185°. On the right iris it is in the same position in zone 5. The right foot corresponds to the right iris, the left foot to the left iris.

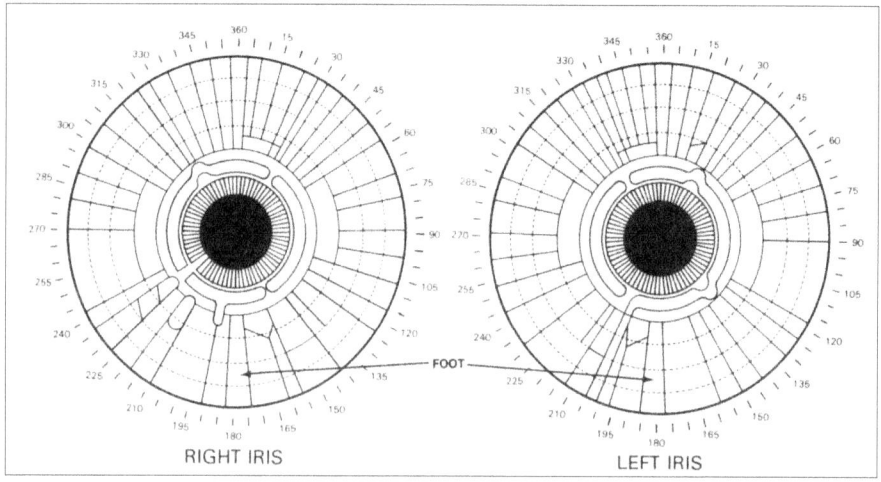

RIGHT IRIS   LEFT IRIS

Athletes foot or fungus can be overcome with pumpkin seed oil and tincture of black Walnut. Plantar warts can be overcome by applying Lobelia tincture and vinegar kept wet on the wart overnight for several nights. Cotton swabs can be kept wet using a plastic bag over the foot kept on with a sock.

Pathologically related signs: leg, heart, colon, male and female organs, cerebellum, knee, and uric acid.

GROIN

The groin is the depression or fold where the thigh joins the abdomen. The groin shows between 183° and 190° on the right iris.

Often the groin area on the iris will look dark to the point that the observer will think it may be cancer. Instead it is usually a hernia were permanent tissue damage has been done to the area.

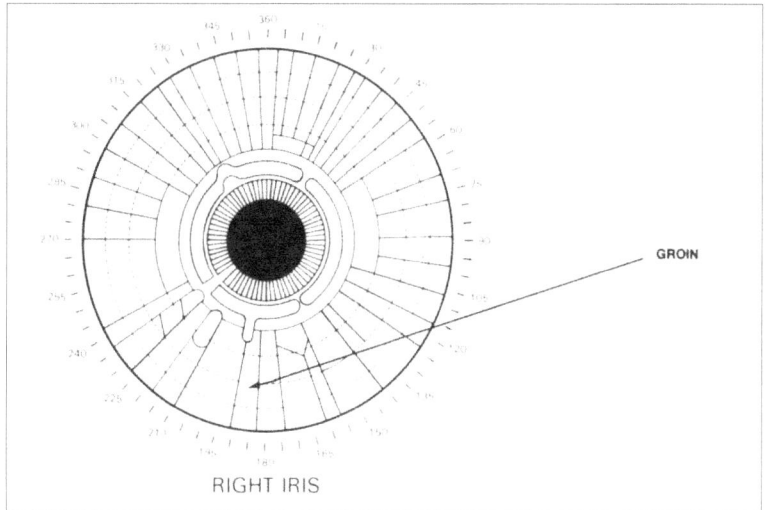

RIGHT IRIS

Hernia is the result of potassium deficiency, causing weak muscle tone. Men usually have weaker abdominal muscles with less stretching capacity and are therefore more prone to hernia.

Pathologically related signs: colon, stomach, appendix, hips, male and female organs.

HAND

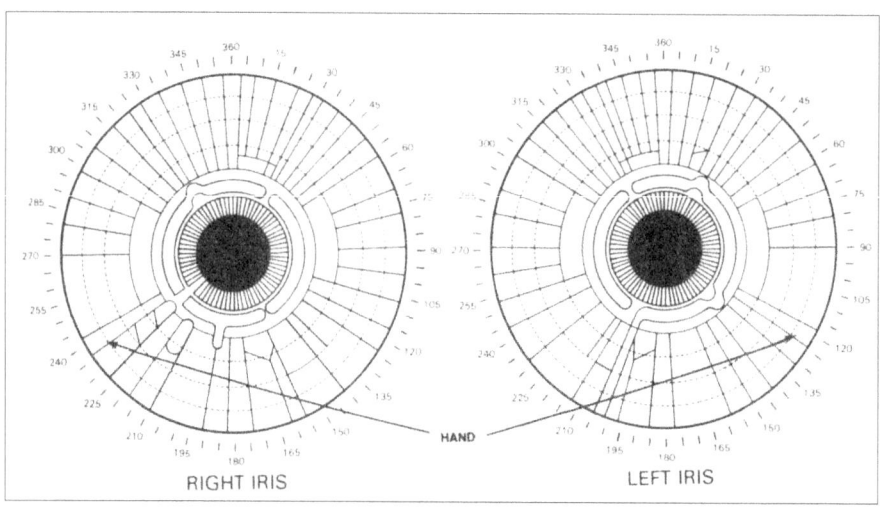

RIGHT IRIS

LEFT IRIS

HAND

Check bony structures for arthritis and permanent damage. Check for dark discoloration of the iris at that point. Hands, like the feet, are subject to warts. (see foot). Fingernails with longitudinal ridges denote a lack of calcium and magnesium. This can also be true if the nails chip or peel.

The hand is that portion of the arm below the wrist that is used for gripping or grasping. The parts of the hand are: the palm, fingers, and thumb. The left hand is found at 120° and 125°, the right hand at 135° to 140°, both in zone 5.

Pathologically related signs: arm, heart, shoulder, submaxillary glands, wrist, and head congestion.

HIP

Since the hip is a major weight-bearing joint of the body it is important to maintain bone structure strength. The hip is subject to many conditions directly related to the continual thrust of body weight either in a sitting or a standing position.

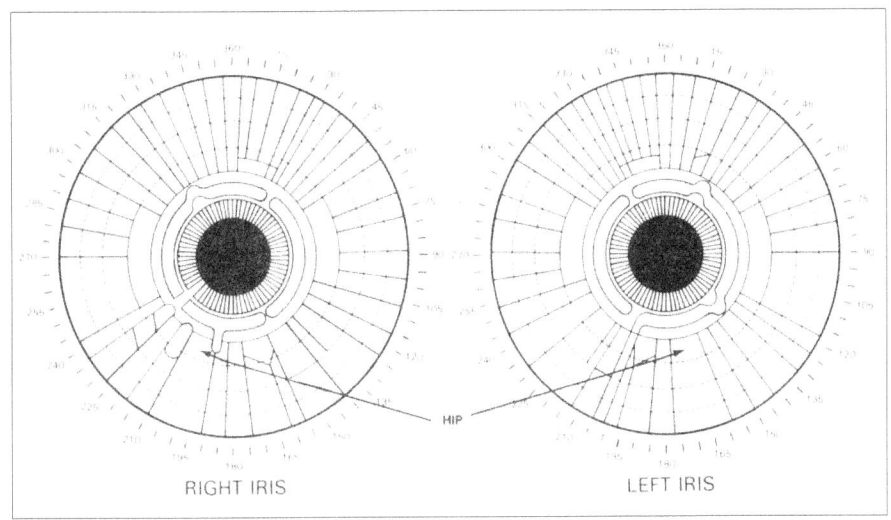

RIGHT IRIS   LEFT IRIS

Congenital dislocation of the hip occurs shortly after birth, resulting from a birth defect abnormality. Girls are more usually affected than boys usually only on one hip rather than both sides. Babies and young children can also experience acute inflammation of the joint usually as a secondary infection such as pneumonia or inner ear infection, so it is important to note white in bony areas of the iris.

Were degenerative arthritis is developing, the area of deterioration will show brown to black, depending upon the kind and extent of the disease. If osteoporosis is developing, the bony area could not only be brown to black but have a pit-like appearance.

The hip is that part of the body including and surrounding the joint where each thigh joins the pelvis. The left hip shows on the left iris between 155° and 175° in zone 3. The right hip between 190° and 210° in zone 3 on the right iris.

A determination must first be made as to the extent and type of deterioration in order to know how to overcome the problem.

Pathologically related signs: continual lower bowel impactions can injure the hips. One short leg, hips out of alignment, or infection such as arthritis or osteoarthritis can cause damage to the hip. Lupus or deterioration of the connective tissues of the body results in bone rubbing upon bone with no cushion between them. Kidney or bladder infections also affect the hip joints. Other related signs are the thigh, groin, and knee.

JAW

Problems relating to the jaw often develop from decaying teeth. Where the jawbone deteriorates it must be scraped. Common sites of abscess formations in the lymph glands, face, mouth or chest can relate to damage to the jaw.

On the iris chart the upper jaw shows the nose as between the mouth, tongue, and lower jaw area. Since the lower jaw shows on the sixth zone, the mouth in the fifth zone, and the tongue in the fourth zone, a very accurate determination can be made as to exactly where the problem exists.

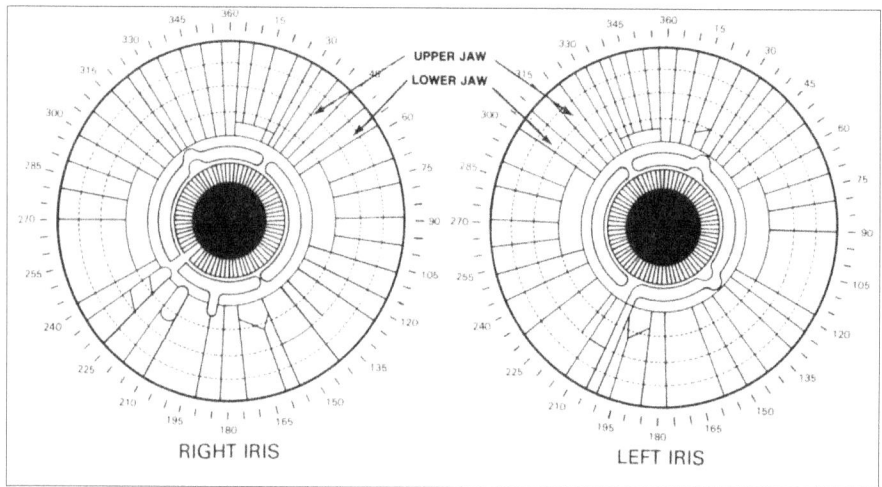

The jaw is the bony part of the mouth that holds the teeth. It consists of two bones: the lower called the mandible, the upper called the maxilla. The upper jaws located on the left iris between 310° and 315°, and on the right iris between 37° and 43°, the lower jaw on the left iris at 302° to 307° and on the right iris at almost 50° to 57°.

When acute signs appear on the iris in any of the above areas, treat as with cold. (See *To Your Abundant Health* under "common cold". See "Acute" and "Chronic" and treat the chronic as with any chronic disease, adding additional calcium as needed.) Chlorophyll is always a good addition to any form of chronic disease, especially in the bony areas. Carrot juice is another excellent addition to the diet in such cases. (See mouth.)

Pathologically related signs: the ears and the submaxillary gland can have a direct effect on the jaw, also the shots given by the dentist can even affect the opening and closing of the jaws. Thyroid, parathyroid, and adrenals have an effect on the jaw. The larynx is also affected by the jaw.

KNEE

The knee is the hinge in the middle of a long limb on the body and is the largest joint. It is therefore exposed continually to injury. After injury, accident, operation or disease, wasting of essential muscles can occur very rapidly if it is not countered by hard, active exercise. No amount of massage, physical therapy, drugs, or even herbs can strengthened the knee muscles – only hard exercise can build up muscles.

RIGHT IRIS   KNEE   LEFT IRIS

The knee is the joint between the thigh and calf portions of the leg. The left knee shows in zone 4 at 175° to 185° on the left iris, the right knee on the opposite iris at the same position.

The knee is subject to inflammation and arthritis. Cartilage damage can trigger arthritis. (See *To Your Abundant Health* under "arthritis".)

Pathologically related signs: hips, ankles, feet, leg muscles, lower bowel, lower spine, and thigh.

LARNYX

The larynx is a structure of cartilage and muscle at the top of the trachea, containing the vocal cords. It shows on the left iris between the tonsils and pharynx almost at 293 degrees, on the right iris the same way only at 65°.

The larynx is the voice box and deals with the expression of sound. The larynx can be changed by injury or infection. Tumors can develop in the area, disrupting voice sound.

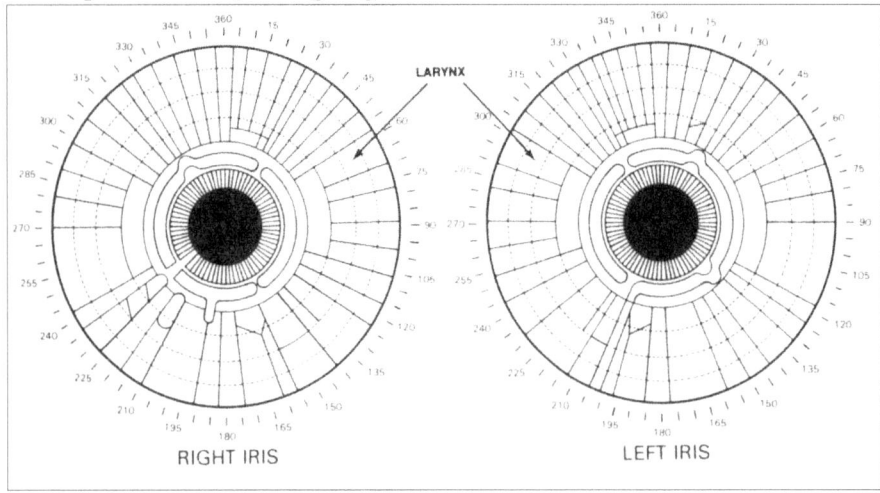

RIGHT IRIS   LEFT IRIS

Pathologically related signs: pharynx, eustachian tubes, tonsils, esophagus, trachea, thyroid, parathyroid, submaxillary glands, mastoid, mouth, jaw, tongue, and bronchials.

LENS

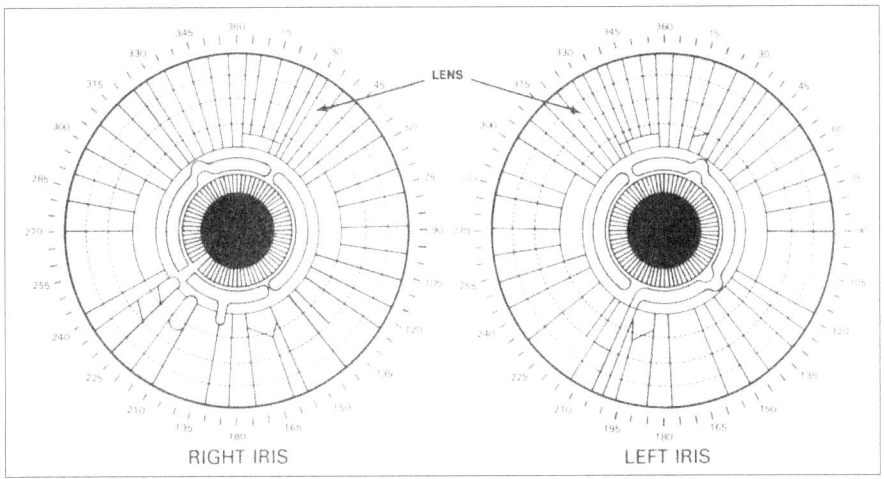

RIGHT IRIS   LEFT IRIS

The lens is that part of the eye that focuses light on the retina. It is transparent and biconvex and is situated between the iris and the vitreous humor of the eye. It shows in zone 5 between 32° and 37° on the right iris, on the left iris in zone 5 between 315° and 323°.

Infection or acute inflammation is treated as with a cold. The herb slippery elm is helpful. Goldenseal root is used as an antibiotic. (See *To Your Abundant Health* under "Common Cold")

The lens can be injured or permanently damaged. The lens can become opaque or clouded, and we call it a cataract. Surgeons have learned how to remove the lens and replace it with a clean plastic lens. Lack of circulation to the head is also a related cause of lens cataract.

The lens can also be cleared with herbs and altered water. General cleansing of the head area is essential to overcoming the problem on a long-term basis by natural lifestyle and mild food diet.

There are some things which may be done to increase circulation to the head area: Correct alignment of the atlas and axis vertebrae, additional calcium in the diet, inversion therapy, and niacin. These treatments have also been useful for both eyes and ears. Carrot juice or vitamin A have been used in connection with other things to strengthen the retina while cleaning the lens.

Pathologically related signs: eye itself, eustachian tubes, ears, general congestion in the head area, brain, atlas vertebrae, axis vertebrae, submaxillary glands, thyroid, and parathyroid.

LUNGS

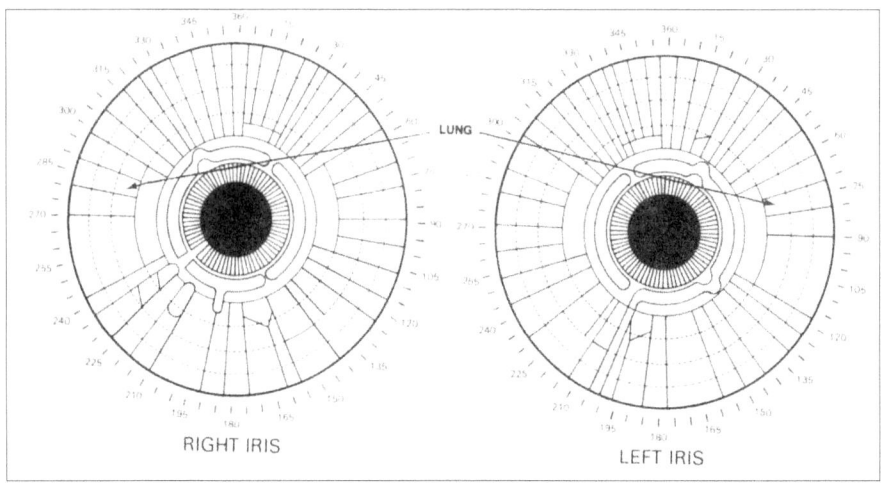

RIGHT IRIS   LEFT IRIS

There are two lungs in the thorax. One is on the left side, one on the right. The lungs are spongy in consistency. Their purpose is to put oxygen in the blood and remove carbon dioxide. The left lung shows in zone 4, 5, and part of 6 between 63° and 90°. The right lung is in zones 4 and 5 between 270° and 297°.

A number of diseases are associated with the lungs: abscess, cancer, tuberculosis, infection, even collapse. Disease in the lungs is very visible on the iris. A determination can even be made as to upper, middle, or lower lung.

Mild food, exercise, and the lung formula herbs such as: mullein, marshmallow, lobelia, comfrey, and slippery elm may be used. Where there is cancer or emphysema, the cleansing formulas are also used.

Pathologically related signs: problems in the lungs are definitely related to toxic waste in the entire body; also the bronchials, breasts, axilla, cerebellum, mastoid, sternum, and heart.

MASTOID

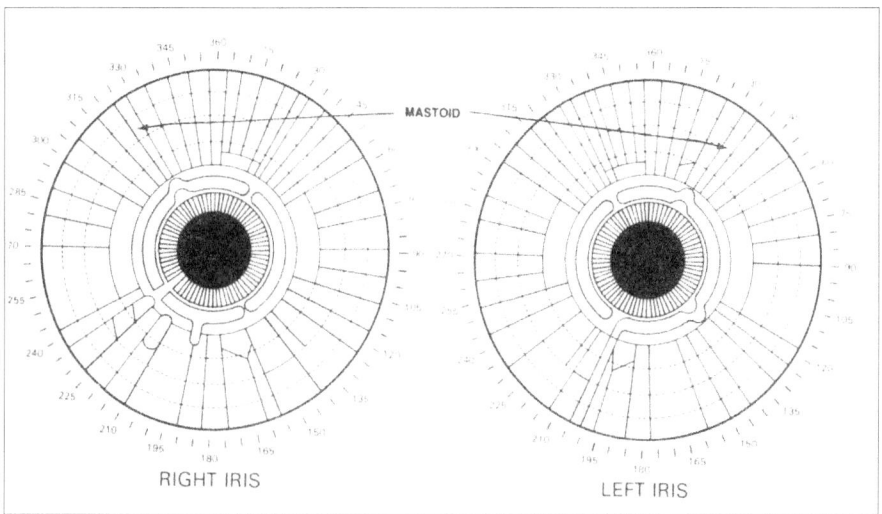

RIGHT IRIS

LEFT IRIS

The mastoid is a projection of the temporal bone just behind the ear. On the left iris it shows between 33° and 40° in zones 3, 4, 5 and part of 6. On the right iris between 323° and 327°, in the same zones as on the left iris.

Mastoid troubles stemming from infections of the inner ear used to be common until antibiotics were discovered. Mastoiditis can eventually cause destruction of bone from pus or infection of brain membranes resulting in fatal meningitis.

Inner ear infections show on the iris as white in the area of the ear and mastoid. A red mask will appear on the skin around the eyes and sockets much like a black eye, only red.

More fruit and vegetables in the diet and no starches, meats, or sugar will ensure permanent changes, and inner ear or mastoid infections will no longer be a problem. Antibiotics will not be necessary. In acute conditions treat as a cold.

Pathologically related signs: nose, head congestion, submaxillary glands, ears, eyes, lungs, eustachian tubes, throat, axilla, bronchials, larynx, mouth, and neck.

MOUTH

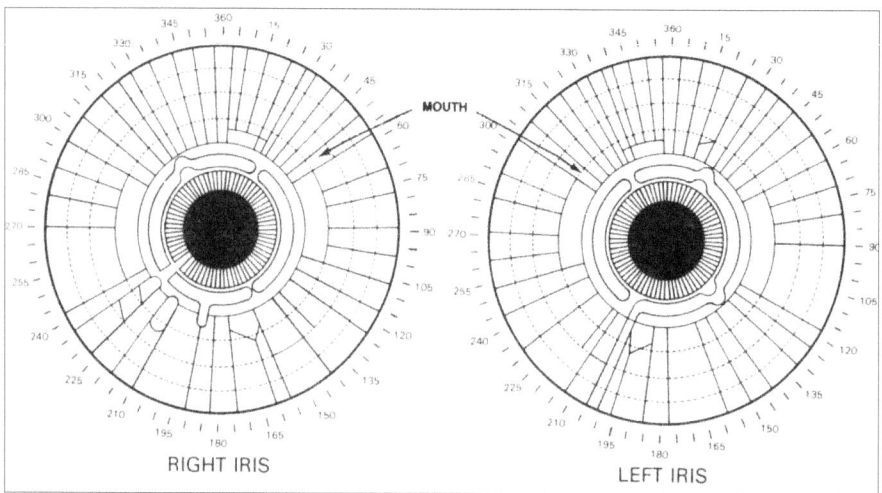

RIGHT IRIS   LEFT IRIS

The mouth is the opening through which food is taken. It contains the teeth and tongue and is the auditory cavity from which sounds are uttered. On the left iris it is positioned between 295° and 305° in zones 3 and 4. On the right iris it is positioned between 50° and 57° in zone 3.

Many diseases are related to the mouth: pneumonia, strep and sore throat, trench mouth, viral mouth and gum disease, pyorrhea, tumor of the mouth, tongue cancer, throat cancer, and canker sores. All could be the result of poor diet, bad oral hygiene or heavy smoking.

A clean mouth is related to a clean and healthy body. Goldenseal and myrrh, equal parts in water as a mouthwash, is healing to all mouth disease, from ulcers to pyorrhea.

Pathologically related signs: teeth, gums, nose, eustachian tubes, submaxillary glands, mastoid, ears, eyes, and larynx.

NAVEL

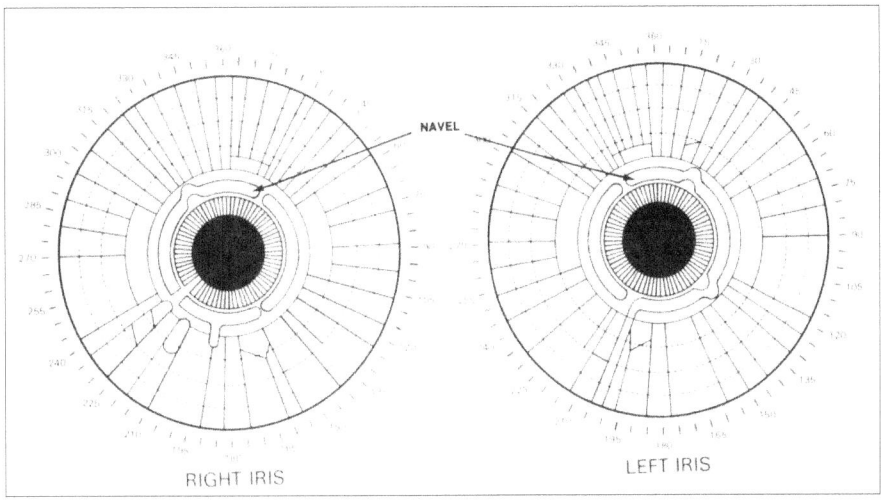

RIGHT IRIS   LEFT IRIS

The navel is a small scar. It is usually a small depression in the middle of the abdomen marking the place where the umbilical cord was attached. On the left iris it is in zone 2 at about 335°, on the right iris at about 30° in zone 2.

The major problem around the navel would be an umbilical hernia (rupture) of the abdominal wall. The greatest danger of a hernia is a strangulated hernia, where so much of the intestines may push through a weak area of the abdominal wall that it becomes impossible to push the protrusion back. The blood supply is cut off and gangrene may set in.

Pathologically related signs: Lack of tone in the abdominal wall and muscles of the body as well as levels of calcium, magnesium, and vitamin C. Children can be born with potassium or other mineral and vitamin deficiencies, because mother had no reserves. Children today are even born with cancer or arthritis. Potassium is the muscle toning mineral and is found primarily in vegetables and fruits. Mothers who live on junk foods, excluding fruit and vegetables, tend to have soft, flabby babies susceptible to hernia.

NECK

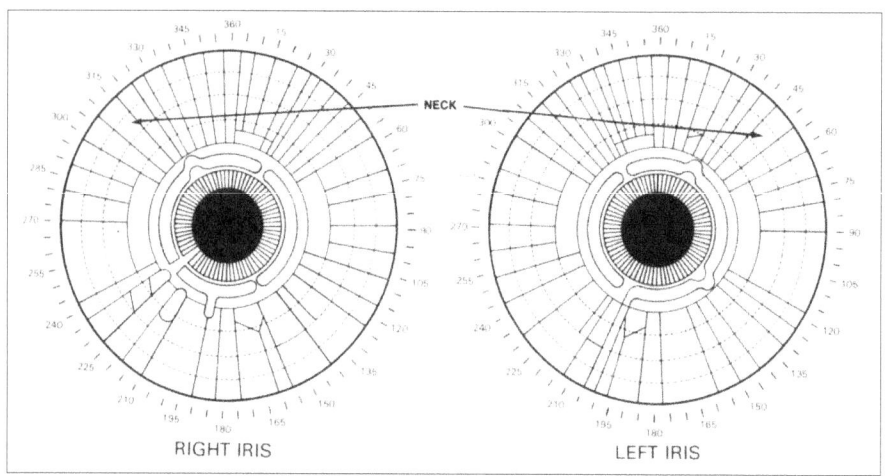

RIGHT IRIS
LEFT IRIS

The neck is that part of the body that joins the head to the body. In iridology it is located on the left iris in zone 5 between 45° and 55°, on the right iris in zone 5 between 305° and 315°

Pathologically related signs: submaxillary gland, thyroid, lymph glands, mastoid, atlas and axis vertebrae.

NOSE

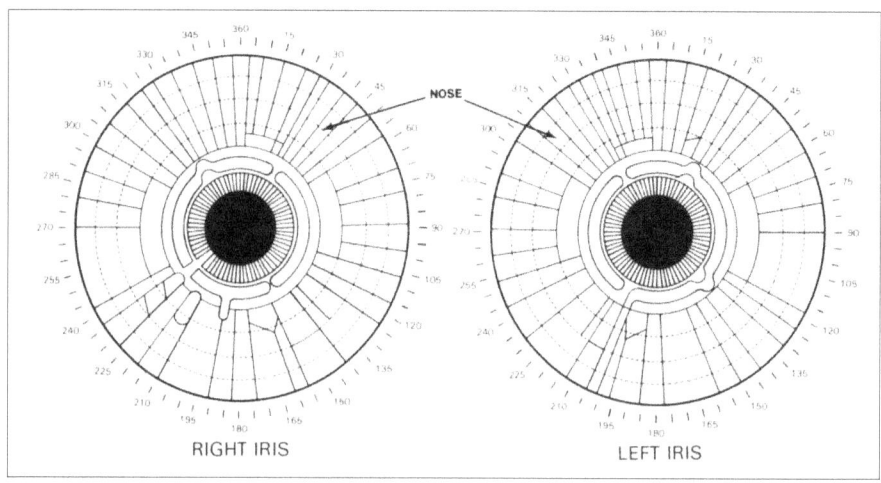

RIGHT IRIS
LEFT IRIS

The nose is that part of the face located between the two eyes and just above the mouth. It consists of two openings for breathing and smelling. On the left iris between 300° to 310°, on the right eye 45° to 50°.

A normal nose is self-cleaning by running or useful blowing. Membrane lining the nose passageways continually secretes what is called mucus fluids by medical science. When disease develops, what is normally called mucus becomes disease and science seems to have no way to distinguish between the terms, normal mucus and disease mucus. Natural healing techniques make the opposite determination and call toxic waste mucus.

A disease almost peculiar to the nose is polyps. A person may change to a mild food diet and cleansing herbs. Polyps will dry up or just fall out like a scab ready to drop off. Cancer or tumors can develop in the nose. Some people are plagued with hay fever or asthma, and when they change to mild food and cleansing herbs their allergies disappear.

Pathologically related signs: headache, head congestion, virus disease, colds, axis and atlas vertebrae, eustachian tubes, ears, eyes, throat, thyroid, parathyroid, and bronchials.

OVARY

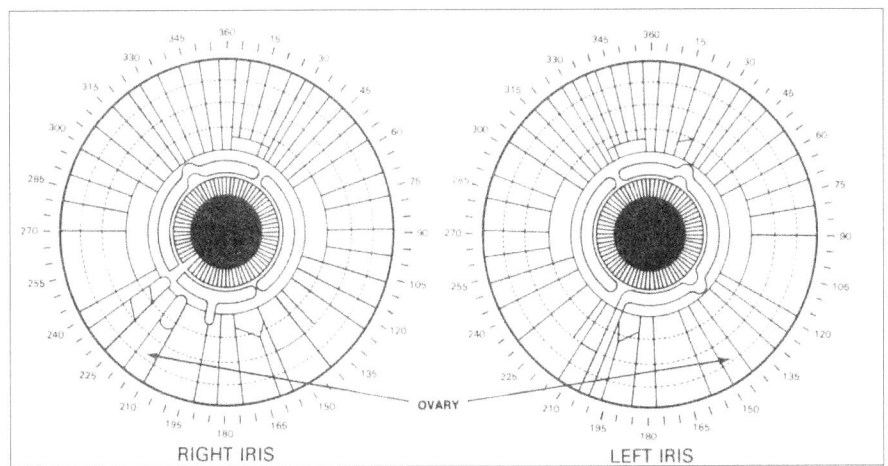

RIGHT IRIS   OVARY   LEFT IRIS

There are two ovary glands in the female reproductive organs. These glands secrete 2 known hormones, estrogen and progesterone which are responsible for development and maintenance of sexual characteristics, preparation of the uterus for pregnancy and ova reproduction, growth of the mammary glands and lactation, along with regulation of menstrual functions. As with all glandular imbalance, note the lines of the iris. Whenever the lines are wavy, check all the glands. If there is anything wrong with the given gland, a spot, lesion, deteriorated lesion or brown spot shows. Spot, line, or lesion will appear on the area of deterioration.

If no such markings appear and the lines of the iris are wavy it is always adrenal stress. (See Adrenal)

The herbs which acts like estrogen are black cohosh and blue cohosh. Black cohosh is the most powerful of the two. The herb which acts like progesterone is ginseng. The minor dysfunctions of the ovaries are related to glands such as adrenals, pineal, pituitary, thymus, thyroid, and female.

The major dysfunctions occur because of cysts or tumors. Elements essential for the normal function of the ovaries are calcium, fluorine, iron, silicon, vitamin B complex and vitamin E.

Pathologically related signs: abdominal wall, breast, colon, foot, and pelvis.

PELVIS

The pelvis is the bowl-like cavity formed by a ring of bone in the rear part of the trunk. It is formed by the sacrum, ileum, ischium, and pubis, and supports the spinal column. It rests upon the legs. This area is also called the pelvic area or pelvic girdle. On the left eye it shows on zones 3, 4, and 5 between 147° and 157°. On the right eye it shows between 210° and 220° in zones 3, 4, and 5.

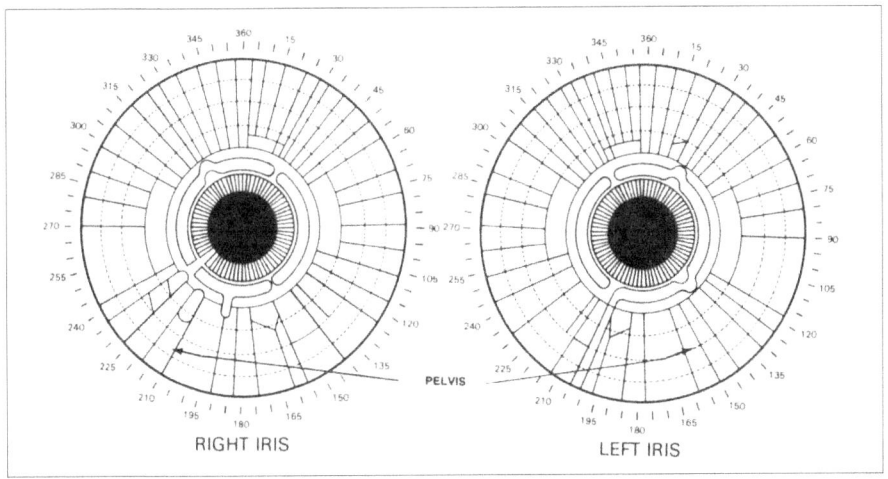

RIGHT IRIS   LEFT IRIS

PELVIS

Because it is associated with reproduction, the pelvis has to support increased amounts of blood, especially during pregnancy, causing a slowing down of intestinal activity. The body seems to compensate by cleansing during pregnancy more than at any other time. If a woman goes on any kind of a good program at all, many diseases can be overcome during pregnancy. Even if a woman does not improve her lifestyle, her body will vomit and cleanse in other ways to compensate. By the time the baby has reached term, a mother on a poor diet may be puffed up with water retention and toxemia.

A break in the pelvis can be extremely serious because it can cause injury to important organs. Infections in the pelvic area are quite common, and there are numerous kinds of infecting bacteria or microscopic organisms which can cause irritation of the skin, painful swelling, itching, gonorrhea, or syphilis. Sometimes warty growths on the skin of the pelvic area may be found. Like all other areas of the body, the pelvic area is also subject to warts.

Cleansing of the entire body is usually the method to overcome even clogged fallopian tubes. Women who could not have children because of obstructions of the tubes have opened the tubes and cleaned out waste and then become pregnant and had fine, healthy babies.

There are various herbs that may be used on skin eruptions. (See *To Your Abundant Health.*)

Pathologically related signs: fallopian tubes, pathological disease in pregnancy, ovaries, lining of the pelvic cavity, skin, and penis.

PENIS

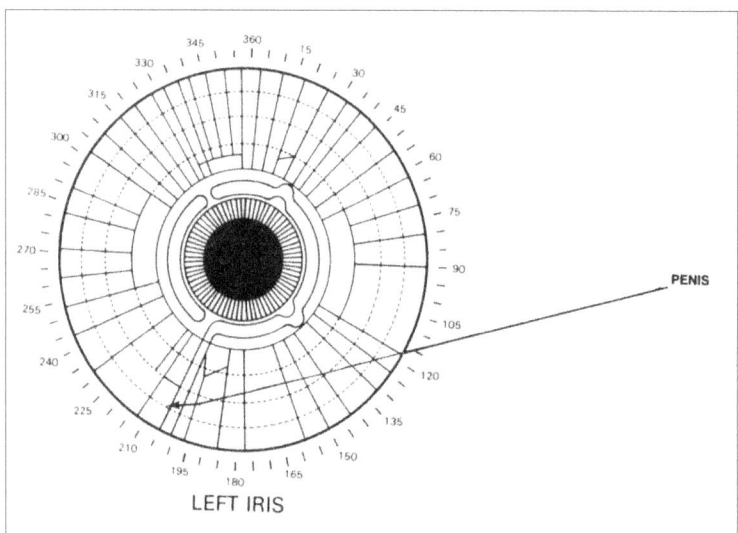

LEFT IRIS

The penis is the male organ of copulation. It is also the organ through which urine is passed. It shows as just past 205° on the left iris only in zones 5, 6, and 7.

Pathologically related signs: pelvis, scrotum, urethra, kidneys, bladder, tumors, lower bowel, testes, prostate, and pituitary.

PERITONEUM

Peritoneum is the serous transparent membrane that lines the abdominal cavity and reflects inwardly at different places to cover the internal organs of the body. The peritoneum is found on both the left iris and the right iris, on the left iris at the outer edge of zone 5 between 150° and 170°, and on the right iris at the outer edge of zone 5 between 185° and 210°.

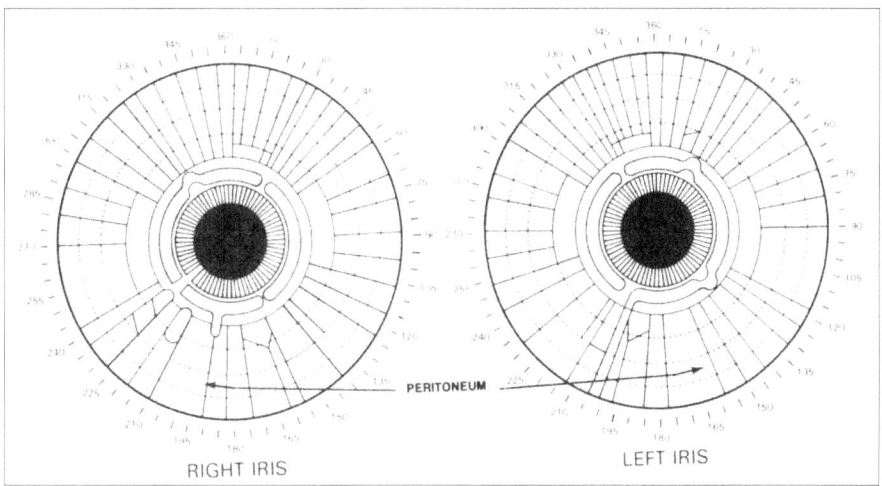

RIGHT IRIS   LEFT IRIS

Malignancies or tumors can develop in the peritoneum or the fat around it without extending out into the colon or small intestines. However, it will eventually penetrate further. Ulcer infections may also occur in the peritoneum. It is interesting how deterioration or acute disease can be so accurately pinpointed in such close proximity's using iridology methods.

Peritoneal deterioration is usually associated with fluid retention in the abdominal cavity. It is important to use kidney herbs and mild food, as well as cleansing formulas, to overcome the problem.

Pathologically related signs: stomach, colon, small intestines, kidneys, adrenals, bladder, liver, spleen, male and female organs, vagina, and rectum.

PHARYNX

The pharynx is the membranous and muscular cavity leading from the nasal passages and mouth to the larynx and esophagus. On the left iris it is positioned between the larynx and the thyroid at the midpoint between 290° and 295°. On the right iris the position is the same, only at about 65°.

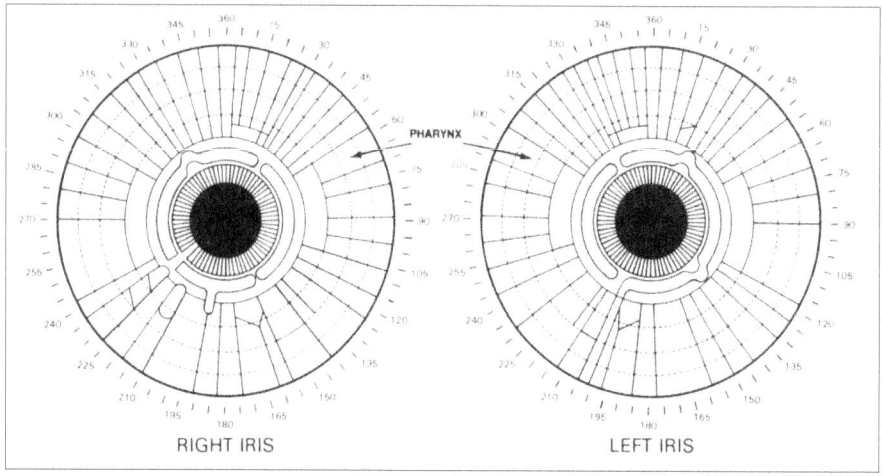

RIGHT IRIS   LEFT IRIS

Pathologically related signs: larynx, esophagus, thyroid, parathyroid, and tongue.

PROSTATE

The prostate is a muscular male gland surrounding the urethra at the base of the bladder. It produces a fluid that is alkaline in nature and is discharged with the sperm produced by the testes. On the left iris it is located in zones 3 and 4 between 205° and 210°. On the right iris it is located between 150° and 155°.

Infections of the prostate are most common in older men, but younger men quite frequently have problems. Diseases such as venereal diseases are contracted by contact. Other infections may be borne by the blood from infections in other parts of the body.

When the lower descending colon becomes impacted and full of parasites, the prostate gland will become swollen, resulting in stoppage of urine. Infections in the prostate may occasionally cause bleeding but most generally cloudy urine and pain. Obstruction of the bladder can be caused by infection in the prostate, tumors, or worms in the lower bowel, which cause constant irritations and swelling. When obstruction of any kind shuts off the bladder's ability to pass urine, life is in immediate danger. About two thirds of all men are believed to have some degree of prostate enlargement.

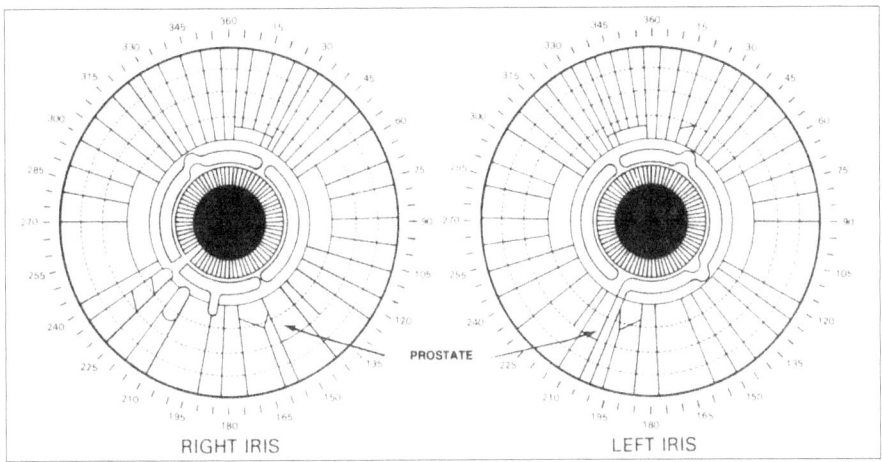

An herbal pumpkin formula will kill the parasites and remove the impaction, along with ginseng tea or ginseng capsules. A quick acting diuretic tea such as buchu will relieve swelling. Every man over 30 years of age would do well to use ginseng. Where there is cancer in the prostate gland it is doubtful that any cancer formulas could cleanse it out in time if the ability to urinate is shut off. If there is little swelling, as in early stages of cancer, the cancer formula, along with herbal pumpkin, has proven to be effective and cleansing out the deterioration in the area and making changes in the iris. Most prostate swelling is relieved simply by killing parasites in the lower bowel and cleaning out pockets of fecal matter in the lower bowel area. Elements essential for maintenance are calcium, fluorine, iron, zinc, silicon, B complex and vitamin E.

Pathologically related signs: kidneys, bladder, urethra, head congestion, penis, lower bowel impactions, scrotum, and testes.

RIBS

The ribs are any of the arched bones enclosing the chest cavity and are attached in the back to the vertebrae. Top seven pair, or true ribs, are attached in the front to the sternum. The left ribs show on the left iris in zones 5 and 6 between 90° and 120°, the right ribs between 245° and 265° on the right iris in zone 5.

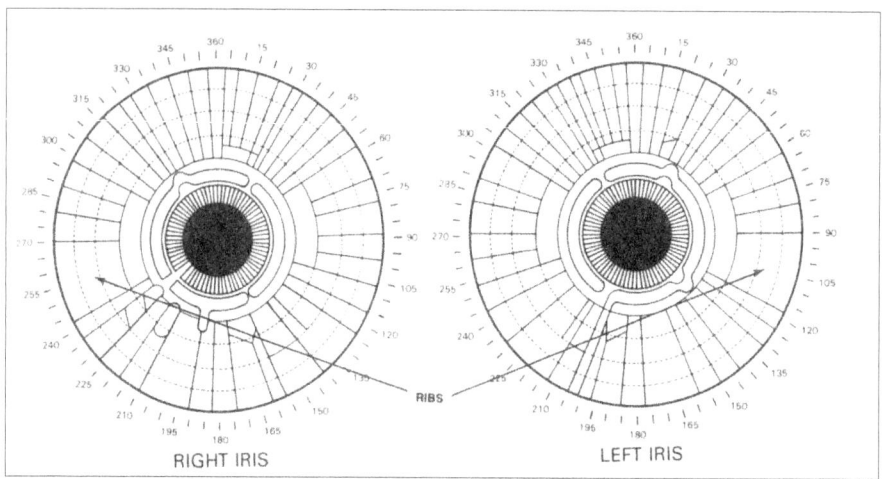

RIGHT IRIS   LEFT IRIS

Broken ribs can be associated with serious puncture, noted by coughing up blood. Breaks show on the iris as lines crossing the normal fiber.

Pathologically related signs: heart, lungs, breasts, pancreas, liver, stomach, kidneys, adrenals, sternum, and thorax.

SCAPULA

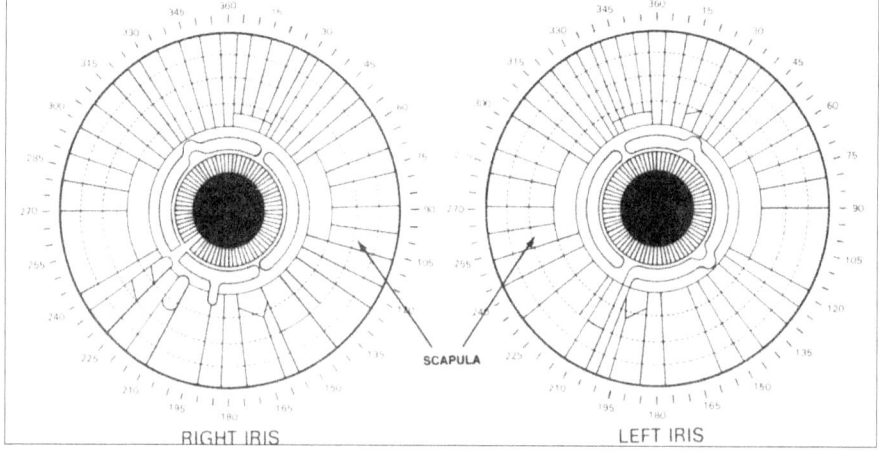

RIGHT IRIS   LEFT IRIS

The scapula is the shoulder blade. It is either of two triangular, flat bones in the back of the shoulder. The left scapula is found in the left iris in zones 4 and 5 between 253° and 263°, the right scapula in zones 4, 5, and part of 6 between 97° and 107°. Markings on the iris in this area are usually associated with injuries. (See Shoulder)

SCROTUM

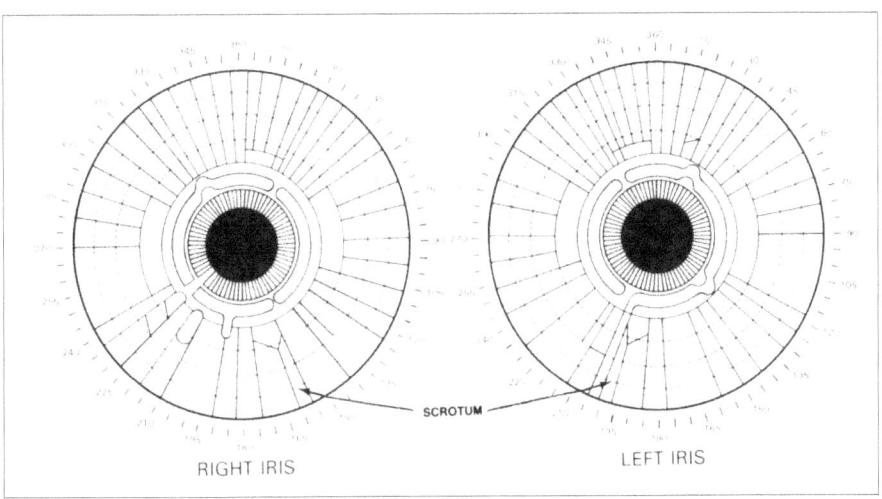

RIGHT IRIS   SCROTUM   LEFT IRIS

The scrotum is a pouch of skin just under the penis containing the male reproductive glands the testicles. These are located on the left iris in zones 4, 5, and 6 between 195° and 200°, on the right iris in zones 4, 5, and 6 between 155° and 160°.

Pathologically related signs: penis, pituitary gland, testes, prostate, urethra, tumors, bladder, lower bowel.

SHOULDER

The shoulder is the joint connecting the forearm to the body. The left shoulder is found on the iris of the left eye at 60°. The right shoulder is found on the iris of the right eye at 305°.

The shoulder is subject to recurrent dislocation and tears in tendons.

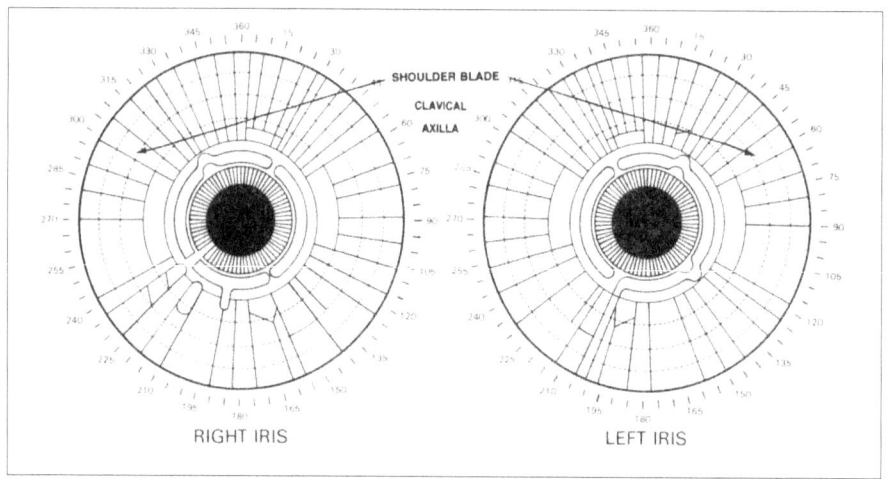

RIGHT IRIS
LEFT IRIS

Pathologically related signs: pain sometimes originates in other parts of the body and causes pain in the shoulder, pain unrelated to the shoulder itself: pleura diaphragm, pericardium, shingles, gallbladder, spinal cord, problems in the neck region, arthritis, muscular dystrophy, bursitis, clavicle, hand, and wrist.

SKIN

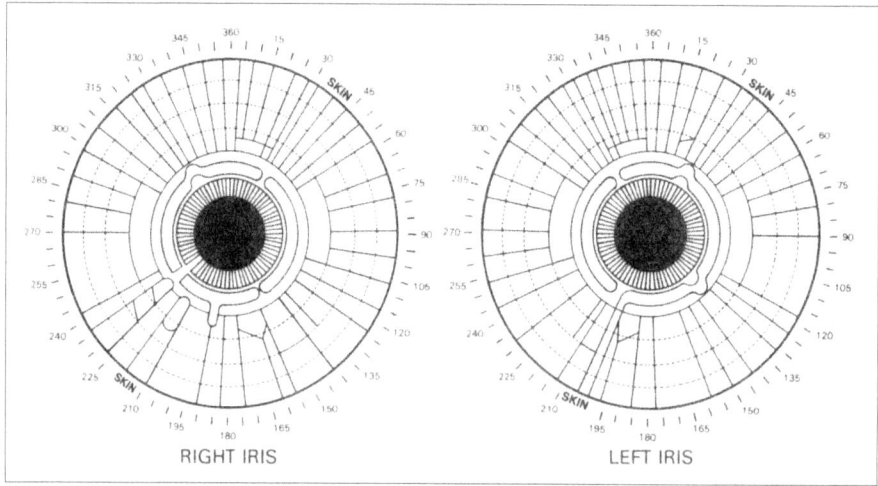

RIGHT IRIS
LEFT IRIS

Skin is the outer covering of the body. The skin contains sweat glands and ducts, hair, a first layer of the skin, a second layer of the skin containing blood and nerves, and the third layer or layer of fatty tissue. The skin is the last zone represented on the iris. It shows in both irises all the way around. Density errors in skin or deterioration are designated in each given area of the iris. For more information on skin see chapter titled SCURF RIM

Pathologically related signs: all of the organs are pathologically related to the skin.

SPLEEN

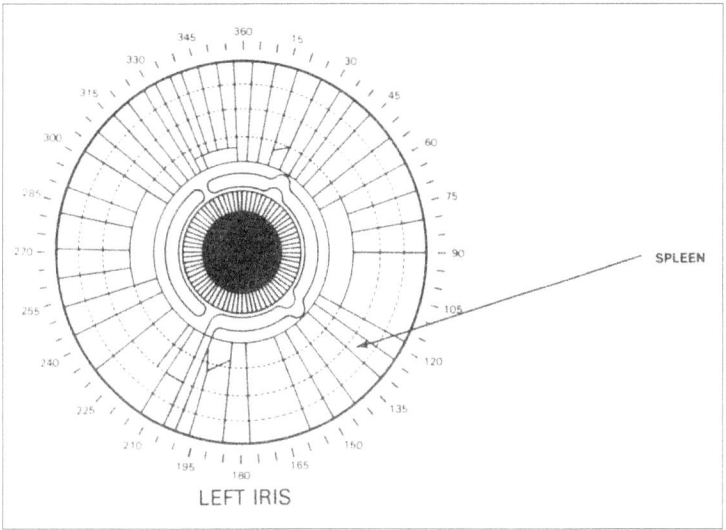

LEFT IRIS

The spleen is a ductless, large, vascular organ in the upper left abdomen near the stomach. Its function is to modify the blood. It is located on the iris of the left eye between 125° and 130° in zones 3, 4, 5, and 6.

A rare viral disease occasionally attacks newborns. This disease is characterized by the enlargement of the spleen. Lymph node enlargement is also associated with the spleen. The spleen acts like the overflow for the lymphatic system until the body can carry off the waste of lymphatic retention. (See LYMPHATIC ROSARY.)

Pathologically related signs: pancreas, duodenum, lymphatic system, thyroid, pituitary, and cecum.

STERNUM

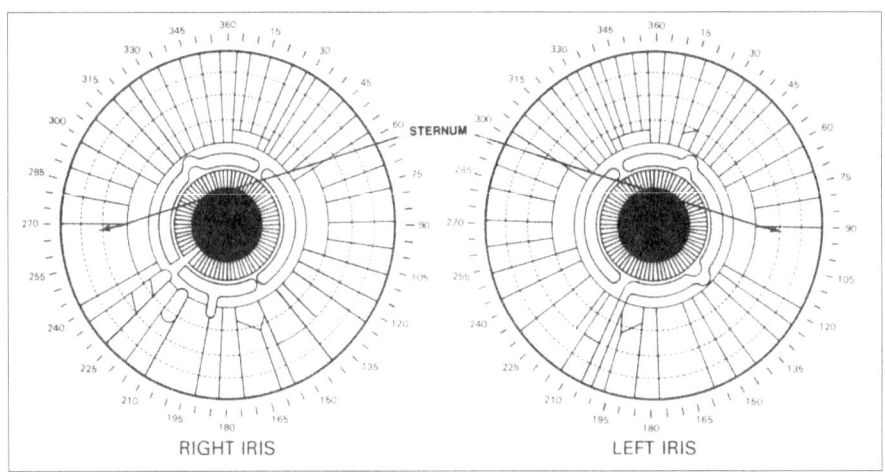

RIGHT IRIS   LEFT IRIS

The sternum is a flat, thin structure of cartilage and bone. The seven major ribs are attached to it in the front of the body. It is also called the breastbone. It shows up at 90° on the left iris, at 207° on the right iris.

Pathologically related signs: ribs, breast, heart, lungs, and thorax.

TEMPLE FOREHEAD

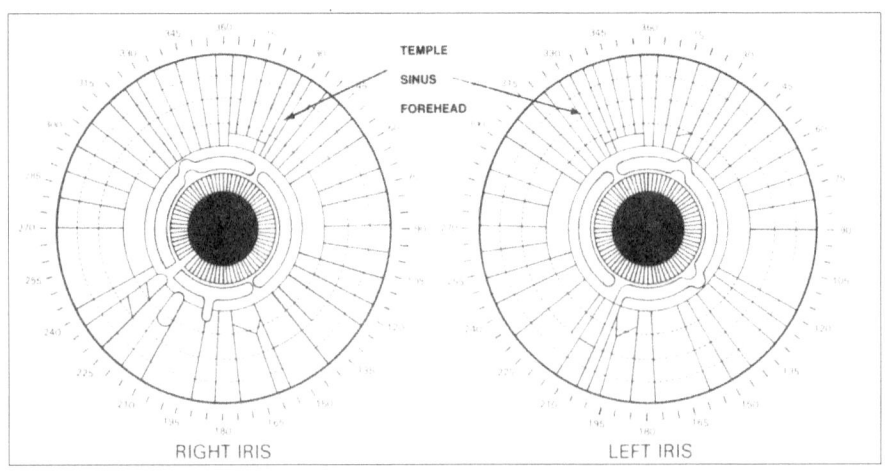

RIGHT IRIS   LEFT IRIS

The temple is either of two flat places or surfaces in front of the ear and behind the forehead. On the left iris it shows between 323° and 327°, on the right iris at 30°.

Pathologically related signs: brain and eyes.

TESTES

The testes are the male sex glands. They are oval in shape and are suspended in the scrotum. They secrete the spermatozoa. The left testicle shows on the left iris between 137° and 147°. The right testicle shows on the right iris between 215° and 220°.

Pathologically related signs: penis, lower bowel, prostate, gland, scrotum, feet, groin, and abdominal wall.

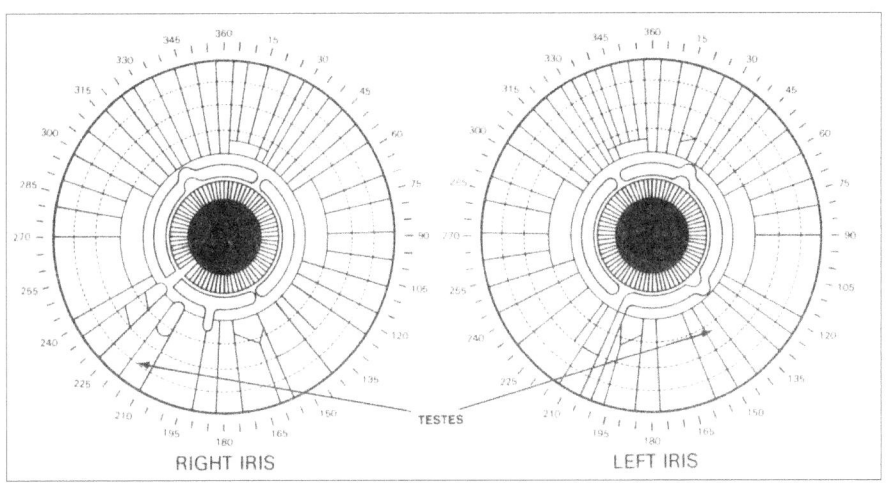

RIGHT IRIS   TESTES   LEFT IRIS

THIGH

The thigh is the part of the leg between the knee and the hip. The left thigh shows in zone 3 at 180° on the left iris, the same is true of the right thigh on the right iris.

Pathologically related signs: knee, hips, and colon.

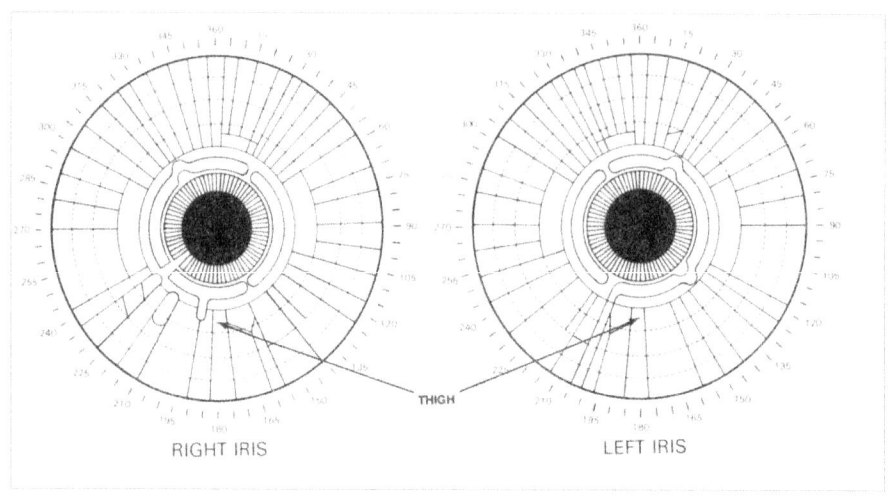

RIGHT IRIS LEFT IRIS

THORAX

The thorax is that part of the body between the neck and the abdomen. The thorax shows on either iris, the left on the left iris at 95° to 105°, the right side between 250° and 260° on the right iris.

Pathologically related signs: sternum and ribs.

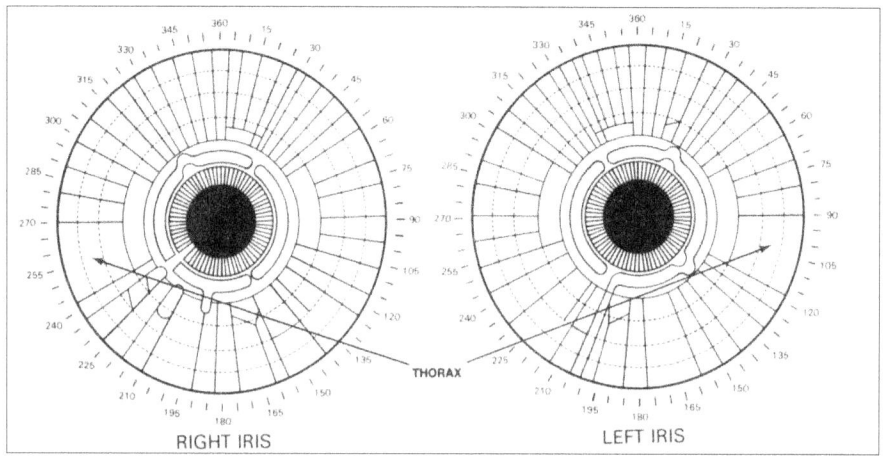

RIGHT IRIS LEFT IRIS

TONGUE

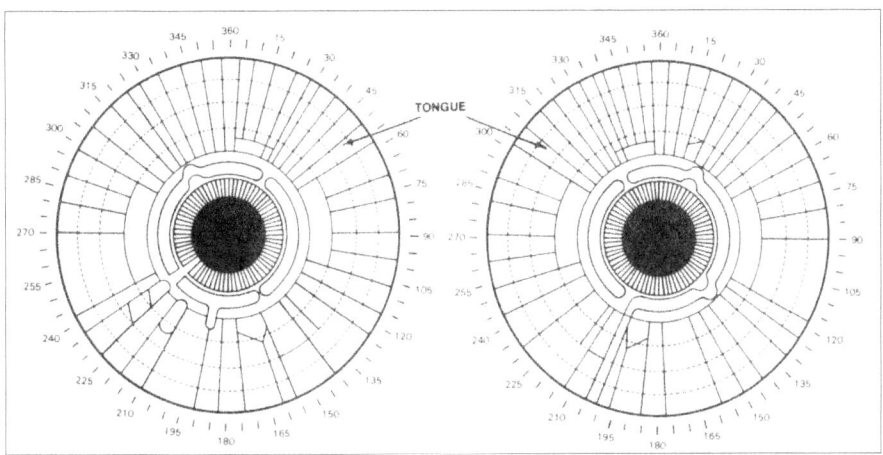

The tongue is a movable muscle attached to the floor of the mouth. It is important in the articulation of speech and the ingestion of food. On the left iris the tongue shows at 300° in zone 5. The tongue shows in zone 5 at 55° on the right iris.

Pathologically related signs: throat, teeth, gums, larynx, pharynx, trachea, and mouth.

TONSIL

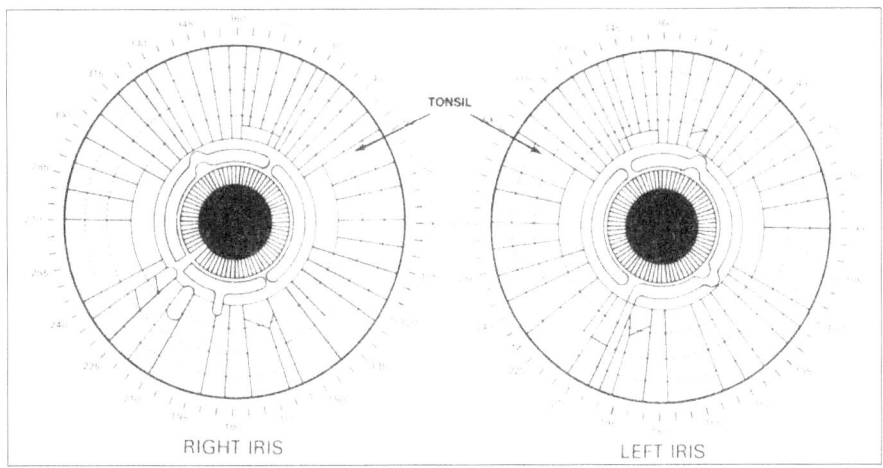

The tonsils are a pair of oval masses of lymph tissue on either side of the back of the mouth that leads to the pharynx. The tonsils protect the body from invading bacteria. On the left iris the tonsils can be found at 295°, at 60° on the right iris.

Tonsils are affected by an acute disease known as tonsillitis. Tonsillitis is not a problem if acute disease is understood (See ACUTE CONDITION). If you are affected by tonsillitis once, chances are it will recur again and again. This recurrence can be overcome by proper diet.

To heal tonsillitis it is a good idea to paint the tonsils with glycerin and iodine mixture every hour. To make the mixture, add drops of iodine to glycerin until it becomes deep Amber in color. When tonsillitis is acute, the most effective treatment is an all fruit diet and to treat the tonsillitis as you would a cold.

Pathologically related signs: throat, submaxillary glands, thyroid, parathyroid, ears, eyes, eustachian tubes, and trachea.

TRACHEA

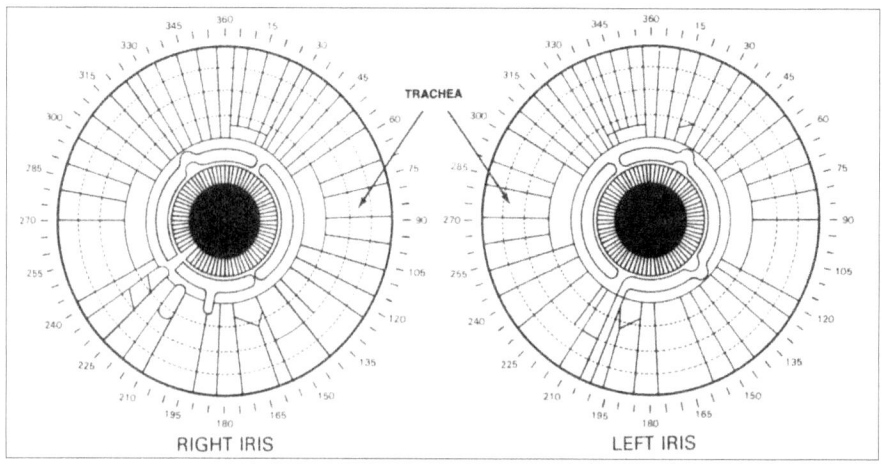

RIGHT IRIS   LEFT IRIS

The trachea is that part of the body which conveys air from the larynx to the bronchi. On the left iris the trachea can be found between 270° and 275°. On the right iris the trachea can be found between 85° and 90°.

Pathologically related signs: bronchials, esophagus, larynx, vocal cords, tongue, and tonsils.

URETHRA

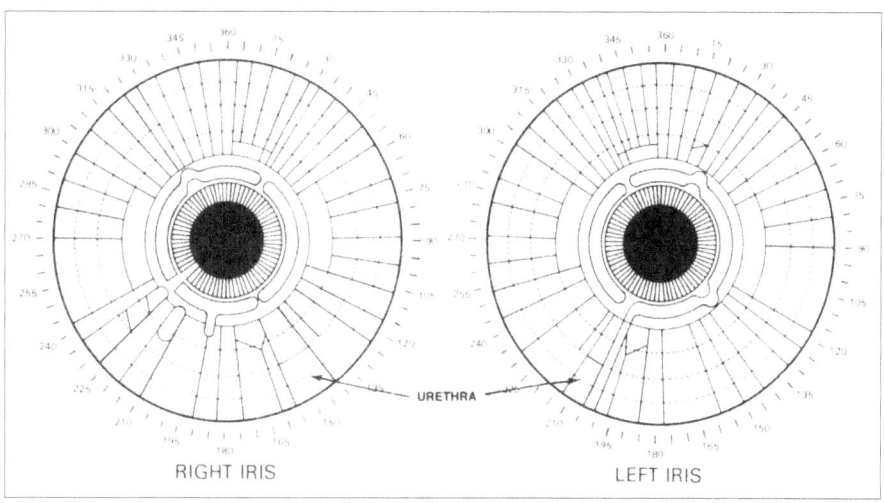

RIGHT IRIS   LEFT IRIS

The urethra is a canal, membranous in nature, through which urine is passed. In a man, sperm is also discharged through the urethra. On the left iris the urethra is found between 205° and 210° in zone 5 and 6 and passing through zone 7, on the right iris between 145° and 155° in the same zones as they left iris.

Pathologically related signs: kidneys, bladder, heart, uric acid, penis, prostate, and scrotum.

URIC ACID

Uric acid is a crystalline acid, the end product of an inaccurate metabolism. It is seen in gout and rheumatism and is caused from gland imbalance, particularly the adrenals. Uric acid can be detected in the left iris between 185° and 190° in zones 5 and 6 and between 165° and 175° on the right iris in the same zones as the left iris.

Pathologically related signs: kidneys, skin, feet, bladder, heart, joints, adrenals, and urethra.

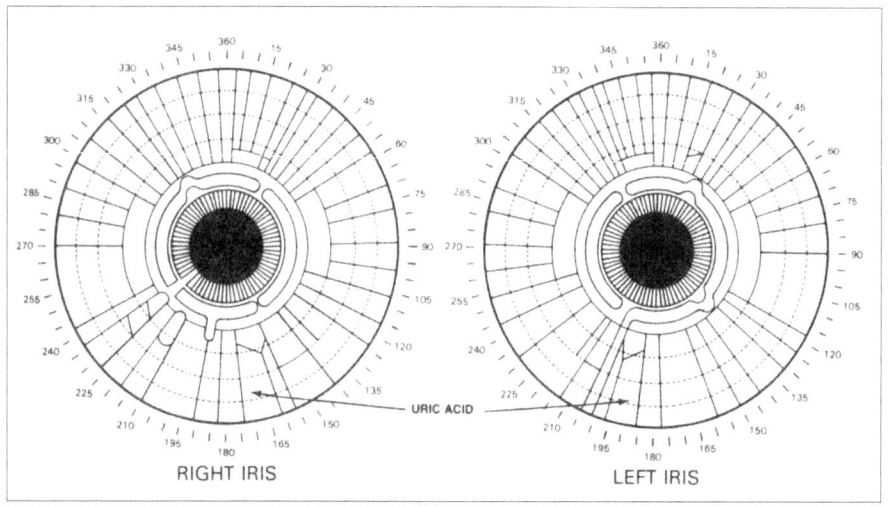

UTERUS

Uterus is a female organ into which the ovum is deposited and where the embryo and fetus are protected and developed. It is commonly called the womb. On the left eye it is found between 205° and 213° in zones 3 and 4. On the right eye it is found between 140° and 155°.

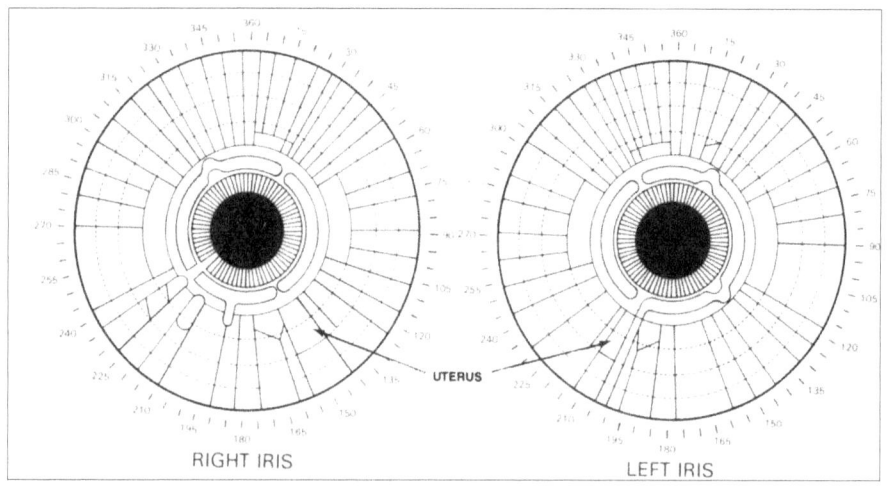

Pathologically related signs: vagina, ovaries, bladder, back, colon, breast, feet, and groin.

VAGINA

RIGHT IRIS   LEFT IRIS

The vagina is a canal leading to the uterus from the vulva. On the left iris it shows between 207° and 213° in zones 3 and 4, on the right eye between 140° and 145° in the same zones.

Pathologically related signs: ovaries, uterus, bladder, colon, rectum, and peritoneum.

VOCAL CORDS

The vocal cords are either of two folds in the larynx, the thicker upper false vocal cords and the lower true vocal cords. Sound or voice is produced by passing air from the lungs passed the lower cords. On the left iris the vocal cord show between 275° and 283° in zones 4 and 5. On the right iris the vocal cord show between 73° and 83° in zones 4, 5, and 6.

Pathologically related signs: throat and mouth.

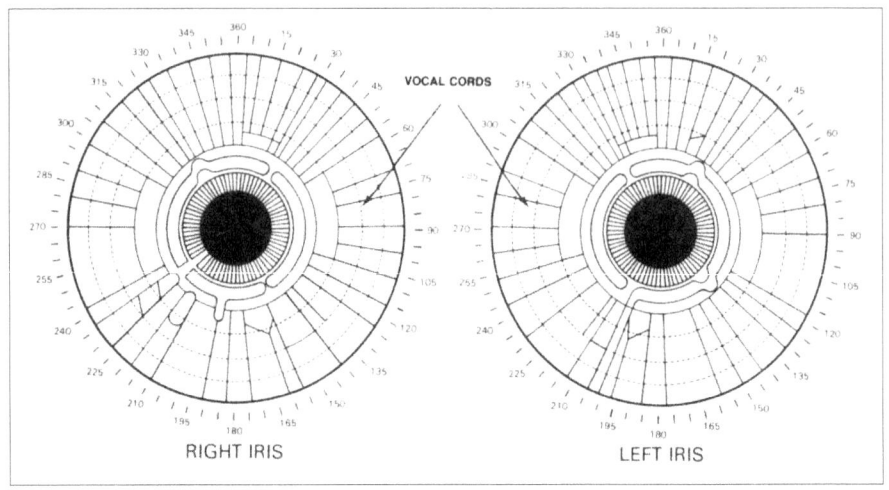

WRIST

The wrist is the joint or part of the arm between the hand and the forearm. On the left iris it is found in zone 4 between 120° and 125°. On the right iris it is found in zone 4 between 235° and 240°.

Pathologically related signs: arm, shoulder, and hand.

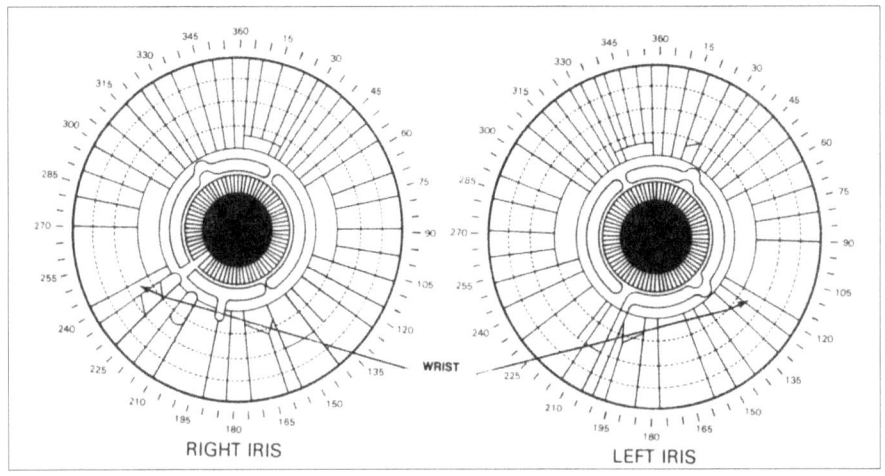

CHAPTER 24

CONCLUSION

High technology's power to treat with an array of techniques, such as keeping a patient alive but offering little hope of recovery, is becoming alarming, proving in the process that daring, surgical procedures and technology have outstripped the body's capacity to heal. With life-support machines, many American patients are caught in medical limbo. Since the dawn of modern medical science fifty years ago to the present time, people have maintained the belief that the sole purpose of medicine was to save life, and the hospital was the place to be saved. However, amazing surgical procedures, coupled with technical advances that could pump blood, breathe, or perform kidney dialysis, have brought with them the dilemma of how to distinguish between life and death. Where do we draw the line? Or quality of life? Doctors, patients, relatives, and the courts are being forced to make difficult and ethical choices in medicine.

Complicating the debate is the escalating cost of so-called health care, which has ultimately been brought about by the cost of technology, as well as inflation. Decisions as to whether to continue trying to keep the patient alive in a limbo situation or pull back and let the patient die are beginning to emerge. The President of the United States has organized a Commission for the study of ethics problems in medicine. It is being forced to make guidelines for such issues as pulling the plug on life support systems, genetic engineering, who will be treated without money, who will be allowed to die when they cannot afford to pay. These are difficult questions, but still another troublesome question forces moral answers regarding the Pandora's box that technology has opened to everyone's view: What about abortion? One wing of the hospital kills babies at 21 weeks, while another wing, a technological or surgical battle goes on to save premature babies. Doctors are now salvaging babies weighing only 2 1/2 pounds, while only 25 years ago a baby weighing only 3 1/2 pounds rarely survived. Nevertheless, a significant number of those premature babies who do survive today, develop physical or mental handicaps. Even with all the great strides that have been made in treating congenital heart defects in premature babies, is the only answer that one mother wants to keep her baby and the other does not? Or is there a moral question to be answered worldwide? Is technology going to continue its onward, upward spiral, continuing to disregard nutrition or the body as a complete mental, physical, spiritual entity? No, it is impossible for this to happen for science is now proving that nutrition does play a major role.

Preventative and holistic medicine have merged out of disenchantment with drugs and the pain of surgery. The promises of drugs could never have lived up to expectation, because they were based on concepts which would change the laws of God and nature. Mankind is now moving out of the pain of a drug oriented culture into a wiser lifestyle, seeking to live in harmony with nature. As man develops a healthier way of life, iridology will play an important role in the prevention of disease.

ZONES OF THE IRIS

RIGHT IRIS

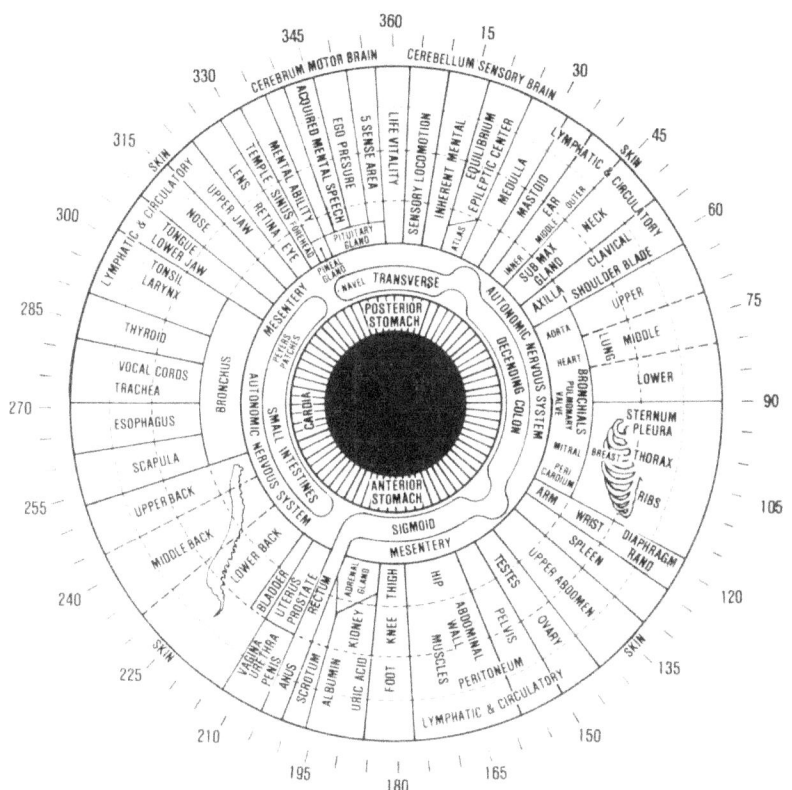

LEFT IRIS

INDEX

EYES

Windows of the Body and the Soul

LaDean Griffin

Cover Photo by Kirsten Tenney
http://adeliaphotography.weebly.com/

DEDICATION

To my father James Melvin Gibby whose philosophy I have added to my own in this book, with love and gratitude for all the truth he taught me and for the example he so lovingly and faithfully set for me.

PREFACE

To write a book on iridology and try to surpass the grand work of Dr. Bernard Jensen would indeed be presumptuous on my part. Dr. Jensen has preserved and popularized iridology for many years with a dedication and love for people, despite heavy pressures, that has been an inspiration to all of us. My purpose in writing this book is merely to add another witness to his work.

In addition, I have learned some things not only about iridology but how to relate iridology with the use of herbs and a mild food diet. The person can not only recognize improvement because of the way he feels but he can also watch the changes as they take place in the eyes. This is a marvel and a wonder to behold, for as the body heals, the eyes change like a kaleidoscope. If such results can be achieved, the logic of a mild food diet and use of herbs must be sound, and iridology must then be a truth.

The use of drugs for healing by established medical methods has too long proven ineffective. It has been previously assumed that drugs were all we needed, and in the beginning the whole idea of finding a wonder drug to solve the world's physical problems met with little resistance. Everyone liked the idea, for it took no effort merely to take a pill and settle all problems. However, thinking people everywhere in the world today have become disenchanted with this idea and the drugs themselves. Mankind is coming to the conclusion that drugs are alien to the natural physiology of man. Medical sciences quest has resulted in failure, for in that quest all the rules and physical laws of the body have been broken. Those who are thinking of looking for alternative solutions are coining a new word – biological medicine – and returning to the herb kingdom for the answers. However, those who are thinking even deeper are recognizing that the real answer does not lie in medicine of any kind but rather in obedience to the laws of nature. Only then will disease flee from us.

IRIDOLOGY

Iridology or iro-diagnosis had its roots centuries ago in ancient Middle East medicine. It has never reached, as far as I can determine, its full potential as a valuable diagnostic tool in the hands of skilled iridologists. Modern medicine with its marvelous optical systems developed the ability to peer through the pupil, revealing the intricate mysteries of the retina, while at the same time bypassing the external, more readily accessible iris. Clinical practitioners today are generally quite ignorant of iridology except for one sign; the arcus senilis. Yet if the doctor's questioned, (How is it that systemis hardening of the arteries shows up in the iris of the eye? How is the iris hooked up, neurophysiologically speaking, to the heart and blood vessels in the limbs?) a blank stare is the usual response. Iridology is not taught in schools of medicine in the United States but is studied, however in some foreign schools, particularly in Germany.

The science of iridology is based upon very precise anatomical and physiological mechanisms which are creator has designed for our use and benefit. Not all are yet ready to accept the concept. But for those who have, iridology has become a wonderful blessing in their lives since these eye-signs are often the first objective changes indicative of a disease process. (You should be aware that pigeon breeders have been depending on eye-signs in their prize racers for many years.)

I am so pleased to write this introduction to this important, new book by my dear friend LaDean Griffin, a most sincere and enlightened lady. LaDean's purpose in her writing and lecturing is to share her knowledge and understanding with her brothers and sisters everywhere, so they might help themselves and their loved ones in maintaining rich, abundant health and promoting healing through natural methods. LaDean has soul and she teaches from the heart, advocating all safe therapies which help our natural abilities in health considerations. Thank you LaDean for a most provocative and challenging volume. Many will call you blessed because of it.

Robert Bliss Vance D. O.
Salt Lake City, Utah
June 2, 1976

TABLE OF CONTENTS

CHAPTER 1

A LOOK INSIDE

Pitifully Poor Politics

It's pitifully poor politics when pretentious politicians and pilfering private promoters purposely prevent or postpone public protection from possible pillage and potential plunder while they painstakingly perpetrate plans for personal plutocracy... What a painful preposterous price the people pay for such pinheaded pigishness

--- And,

As long as we tolerate such black and blighting blunders we'll continue to be in the red. So, for freedom sake and our own, let's be Real, United Americans in Our United States.

J. Melvin Gibby 1964

**Think
America First!**

Aside from the fact that people get better on my programs, of all the subjects I teach, iridology is probably the study which proves my theories more than any other single thing. As people watch the change for the better in their general health, they are amazed to watch the changes taking place in the iris of their eyes. It is both a thrilling and almost magical transformation that occurs; an exciting new demonstration of the art of healing – or at least it is new to modern man. Iridology: the practice of analyzing the inside of the body by the iris of the eyes. It dates back to the 12th century, and has probably been known by some great physicians as far back as the beginning of time.

My purpose is to teach some of the main things to look for and how to use herbs, mild foods and vitamins in conjunction with what is discovered in the eyes. The study of iridology could be an important facet of your life. We have been presented with a grave spectacle of physical degeneration increasing daily around us as a result of fear tactics through the wide use of drugs. It has not been without reason that these dire results have caused such general dependence upon the doctor.

As we have watched the jubilation over the wonder drugs sink into the decay of degenerative disease they cause, we can see that to try to find the answers ourselves, when it is almost too late, is a lonely ordeal.

Reading through an old book on iridology dated 1924, I suddenly thought that the medical doctor who wrote it had never in his wide experience ever seen the kind of eyes we see today. The eyes we see today since 1924 and the 50 year use of drug therapy, look shattered, filled with all manner of degeneration not known in 1924. We even see in the photos taken in my class is the most seriously degenerative diseases of old age showing upon the eyes of babies and young children. Another 50 years of drugs and we will not have to worry about the population explosion. On the contrary we will have to worry about taking care of all the blithering idiots and sick old babies we will create in future generations. We now have more retarded or maimed children or children with birth defects than ever before in history. The proportion of Americans wearing glasses has also increased. Then we have the audacity to proclaim the great advances of medical science. Thinking people everywhere are searching for alternative solutions to their health problems and finding them among the natural, simple and inexpensive medicines God has provided in the herb kingdom. Medicine rip-offs by doctors and pharmacists are costing the United States taxpayers $3 billion a year, says a recent newspaper. But what about the rip-off that inevitably occurs through our being a drug oriented society? What about the drug caused diseases we contend with today? An article came out in a Los Angeles paper by a large medical hospital which is trying to overcome the problems of errors made in giving medication. It said that the average doctor is only familiar with a tiny percentage of the 7000 principal drugs in the medicinal arsenal. As a result, wrong dosages and wrong drugs are used. It was stated that 100,000 serious errors are made daily in American hospitals in preparing, prescribing and dispensing medications. It was further stated that these mistakes are causing the deaths of thousands of hospital patients every year. Many patients are dying who don't need to die, and others are not recovering rapidly enough because of the errors and not receiving proper medication for their disease. Their reasoning was that the method to help correct the errors was close security programs to safeguard against nurses, doctors and pharmacists making these errors.

Virchow said:

"Some doctors make the same mistakes for 20 years and call that experience."

Not only do we have a concern about misuse of drugs but we also have a concern about the drugs themselves. In addition, we have the dangers involved in the use of over 3000 different chemicals being used in the distribution of commercial food products, many of which are suspected of being harmful. Some have been proven to be dangerous or at least suspect, says the Plain Truth magazine. Coal tar dyes are suspected of being harmful to man in nearly any amount if continually consumed. We see headlines warning us continually, such as, "Rat livers injured by color dye," "Cancer inducing chemicals added to food for humans," Specialist says "Britain bans treated fruits from U.S."

Four to five hundred totally new chemicals are put in our food each year. What about the potential long-term hazards? Many articles are finding their way to the public about the poisons in our food and thinking people everywhere are becoming deeply concerned.

Cyclamate alone has been contained in 172 brands of products with an annual sale of about $1 billion. How many more poisons do we unwittingly consume?

Because of the controls of the FDA on drugs, natural herbal formulas are restricted by the medical monopoly on drugs, and yet herbs are not drugs per se. What about the FDA's control of all these new chemicals finding their way into our food supplies with no apparent restriction or control? Who is running this country: the scientists, the FDA or the people? A man who has been helping leper cases with herbs, with some startling results, was stopped by the FDA. He wrote to the president, dated November 17, 1973:

Dear Mr. Pres.:
Today is the 4th anniversary of our being closed by the Food and Drug Administration. Although we asked them to make an appointment for a demonstration, and showed them some 200 or more letters from our clientele, my wife and I could see that they were not interested. They said our letters could be phony. We asked them to select as many as they liked, and call them anywhere in the country on our telephone. He then stated, it is too late! I wanted to know why, as it is never too late to cure cancer. He said, now listen to me and to what I have to say, and I will only say at once, Mr. Crosby. From now on you are closed, and if you send or ship your product over state lines, you face IMPRISONMENT! At 70 years of age, it was an extremely difficult thing to accept, having your income suddenly stopped, without a chance to prove anything to anyone, (especially, after all the mistakes the FDA have recently made) is making a farce out of "FREEDOM OF FREE ENTERPRISE!"
Our formula will cure cancer in any form, even tumor of the brain. It contains NO DRUGS, it is NON-TOXIC. Our formula will cure MELANOMA completely in just 14 days. When a patient has melanoma, the physicians tell the patient, there is no use for surgery, they have from 45 to 60 days left. This is not necessary, and we implore you sir, for

12

an appointment, so that we may show you the efficacy of our formula.

BREAST CANCER can be cured in 60 days without surgery, without drugs, chemicals or injections. Think Sir, what this would do for WOMANHOOD, throughout the entire world!

Trusting we will hear from you in the near future, I remain Sir,

Sincerely yours,
Kirley Crosby

This is the kind of answer Mr. Crosby receives for his inquiries:

May 4, 1971

Dear Mr. Crosby:

The White House has forwarded to us for reply your letter of March 11, 1971, concerning your formula for cancer.

If you propose to offer your formula for import into this country, you should understand that it must comply with the federal (U.S.A) Food, Drug, and Cosmetic Act. Enclosed is a publication which described in non-technical terms the requirements of the Act.

We believe your formula may be a "new drug" as that term is defined by the Act. A "new drug" is a drug which is not generally recognized among qualified experts as safe and effective for its intended purposes. A "new drug" may not be distributed in interstate commerce in this country, or imported into this country, until its sponsor has submitted to us, and we have approved, a new-drug application containing substantial evidence (i.e., evidence based on adequate and well-controlled investigations, including clinical investigations) which establish that the drug is safe and effective for its intended uses.

The data to be submitted in support of a new-drug application must be based on the type of testing described in Regulations 130.3 and 130.4 of the enclosed copy of the New Drug Regulations.

Sincerely yours,
Donald N. Kilburn
Assistant to the Dir.
Division of Case Guidance
Office of Compliance
Bureau of Drugs

Pictured on page 58 is the leg before herbal treatment and after treatment.

There has to be a better way than such things being restricted by the powers that be. How soon will the people awaken and take back the rights from these powerful monopolies? The movement is on and we can see such a wave of health articles not known since the Vitamin craze of the 30s. People are taking a long hard look at the high cost of dying. Books are being written and movies pan the hospitals and doctors. People are studying and are not so willing to allow the doctor to rule them every waking moment. People are learning to take care of themselves and finding out that they can. The new thing is learning how to take care of yourself and keep yourself well. This is called preventive medicine, a popular new phrase that has been coined out of the struggle.

Many years ago Leah Widtsoe wrote:

"It is noble to help those who are ill and suffering, while trying to restore their health, but it is far nobler to teach one or a thousand how to build and maintain health so that suffering and disease may be prevented."

In a letter to the Mormon Battalion dated August 19, 1846, Brigham Young said:

"If you are sick live by faith and let the surgeon's medicine alone if you want to live, using only such herbs and mild foods as are at your disposal."

The newspapers as far back as 1972 state that more than 3 million persons needlessly undergo surgery each year, 36,000 resulting in death. On the other hand, a San Francisco paper says the organic food business has increased to such a phenomenal rate that there is now a far greater demand than supply of such fruits and vegetables. When worldwide health series are also beginning to emphasize disease prevention and articles such as those which came out in the "London Times" recently began to agree with some new health ideas. But scholars and doctors will probably bull-doggedly hold onto tradition. As an example, recent radio talk show interviewing such a person showed the sorry predicament of an information school-computed individual who had no ability to reason things out for himself. It seems that the young lady asking the questions was deliberately asking all the key questions against natural methods, using every few minutes this man's degrees to prove he knew all the correct answers. As the questions and answers continued one could feel his confusion, could see his complete stupidity about natural health methods. He kept saying, "Be sure to see your Dr." whenever he got in an awkward corner. He seemed to know that vitamin C helped but stated that all other vitamins were unnecessary. After stating that we should just eat a well-rounded diet and take our chances at getting all the vitamins, someone asked him about organic gardening. At this time he proceeded to say that organic fertilizers were haphazard, that the chemical fertilizers could be planned. He also stated that there was no harm in stilbesterol-fed animals if the animals were butchered correctly. This is the kind of inconsistent and stupid answers we get among the computed scientist or doctor who finds his boat rocking because of the evidence all around him. He somehow has to argue in defense of the errors he has computed because it would suddenly put him in a category of the unlearned if all this information he has spent so much time and money accumulating were suddenly to be proven incorrect. As I have stated in my other books, the physician today must use only the chemicals listed in the Physicians' Desk Reference or he is not allowed to practice. The FDA controls any additions to the book, leaving us all wondering who is controlling what. It seems that if it is a chemical, no matter how harmful it may be, it somehow gets passed on to public use, but if it is plant derived, such as Laetrile or like the herbs Dr. Meyer was using for leprosy or DMSO, it is impossible for it to get to the public market.

One of the great herbs discovered in the last decade for pain Dimethyl Sulfoxide or DMSO, has been held back by FDA since 1960. It is made from the cement substance of trees, which puts it in the herbal class. Therefore, it is unacceptable. DMSO has been used on 50,000 patients, but that is apparently not enough. These are some of the things, discovered in tests, which Dimethyl Sulfoxide, DMSO is helpful for when made from a natural substance:

Retarded children
Brain-damage
Analgesia
Anti-inflammative
Muscle relaxant
Diuretic
Increases antidotes
For soft tissue injuries
Peyronie's disease
Acute epididymitis
Regressive growth influence
Used in veterinary medicine
In angina prevents damage to heart muscle
Brain and spinal injuries in animals
Controls inflammation
Reduces pain
Burns
Arthritis
Pain of broken bones
Clears up gum conditions
Disc disease pain
Clears up inflammation and wipes out infection in decayed birth
Skin transplant – no scar – fracture, pain, swelling

If a person drinks liquor after treatment, the DMSO increases alcohol and causes drunkenness with only 2 drinks. A sprained ankle can be healed in 3 days instead of a week making it very useful for athletic injuries.

One thousand two hundred articles on DMSO have appeared in medical journals all over the world. It was approved in Germany and

Austria in 1965. It is now being synthetically made from coal tar and petroleum in those countries. We as a people have allowed laws to be passed which have boxed us right into a corner. We have allowed politicians and the bureaucracy to make laws which take away all of our freedoms, how can we progress? How can we learn anything new? How can we reevaluate old truths to our benefit? If these laws remain and lack of respect, causing uncertainty about existing medical methods continues with mounting costs, people could slip back into old superstitions as has been done many times in history. Whether or not medical science will openly acknowledge its failures with drugs, grievances toward the medical world are beginning to build to a national sentiment and will one day be more than a joke on TV or a movie that pans hospitals. It will culminate in a bitter contest where medical science will finally rule and people will drift off into suspension. Or natural methods will win and scientists who have held onto their computed information will stand red-faced, exposed to the truth. Before we take a look inside of the body through the iris of the eye, we need to take a good look inside our country's medical practices and find out just why iridology is not accepted.

When men like Dr. Lyman Smith of Elgin, Illinois, Dr. V. Mooney of Downey, California, orthopedic surgeon, Dr. Joseph E. Brown who wrote in Clinical orthopedics about the enzyme chymopapain, made from papaya and Dr. Charles Hech, Executive Director of the American Academy of orthopedic surgeons in Chicago, all speak favorably for the enzyme for helping back disc problems and are still not able to get past to the FDA to help with the treatment made of papaya fruit and when Dr. Krebb, who made Laetrile out of apricot pits has the same problem, is there something or someone who is trying to keep us from the wonderful discoveries to be found in biological medicine and hold us bound to the side effects of drug therapy, could we be beginning on the last struggle of a weakening dictatorship which is losing power with the people because it does not get the job done?

As we watch what has happened over the past 50 years of drug therapy in changes in the average iris as compared to the things earlier iridologists saw, we begin to understand the magnitude of corruption and inefficiency which has been a plague rather than a progression. As you begin to understand iridology, you will find a whole new world of wonderful but horrifying truth opening to your consciousness. You will begin to realize that you can no longer relinquish the responsibility of your body to the care of another person but you will also learn that preventative medicine and know-how is a supreme asset.

CHAPTER 2

THE METHOD

In order for iridology to be of value to the layperson so that he may be able to analyze the inside of his body, it would also be essential to understand how to use iridology in conjunction with herbs and correct diet in a specific way. This chapter is designed to do just that. It is not my intention to teach all facets of iridology but rather those essentials which will help each person to help himself after determining from his eyes those things which are wrong. The eyes are the windows of the body. Every error, injury or pathological disturbance which takes place in the body finds its way to the windows, where we can peer in to discover the uttermost dark, secret and hidden places. As the body heals through correct principles, the eyes will change like a kaleidoscope, a wondrous miracle to behold.

In my books, *Is Any Sick Among You?* and *No Side Effects*, fasting, the use of mild foods, correct food combinations, home remedies with herbs and vitamins, and care for the colon are discussed. The layperson will now learn to be specific in determining what is wrong in the body. To learn iridology, without learning what to do for what is seen, would be of little value to anyone other than to play parlor games, and such games could hurt more than they could help. As we begin to take our first look into the body, we need a good eye loupe and flashlight in order to see.

To see one's own eyes, use an eye loupe directly against the eye and a magnifying mirror in a bright light. A darker shade than the color of the eye will manifest itself as an outline on the colon, stomach, autonomic wreath and periphery, or outside, line of the iris.

Anything other than these darker lines in any way shape or form showing on the iris of the eye is disease or inherent weakness. When it is inherent weakness, there will be a darker shade than the color of the eye, either in a shadow or a bowed-out place which we call a lesion.

(1) **TEXTURE** See Picture Page 46

If the texture of the iris is like fine silk, the body is inherently strong. If it is loosely woven with these darker shadows showing in between, whether in a lesion or a shadow, this shows inherent weakness in the area where the darkness occurs. We can determine by this, the body's strength and ability to heal. The finer the texture, the better the ability to heal.

(2) **FOCUS LINES** See Picture Page 46

Sometimes we may see an older person whose texture is excellent and yet the lines of the eyes have become flat rather than sharply in focus. This indicates that the body had a good inherent health but is growing old. On the other hand, you may see a young person who has a sharp focus of the lines of the eyes but a loose texture. This young person could have more strength than the old person even though he may be inherently weaker. His body will not last as long or remain as well as long as the older persons whose body has had fine texture. A young person can have a flat focus and a fine texture merely showing weakness. When a young person has a flat focus and a loose texture the weakness is compounded. The first thing we look for is inherent strength of texture.

(3) **THE HEART** See Picture Page 46

The next thing we look at is the heart. There should be no marking of any kind showing on the iris in the heart area unless there is something wrong.

As far back as 1964, cardiovascular diseases killed 921,500 people in the United States annually. When the prophets have said that in the last days men's hearts will fail them, it appears that we are living up to latter-day expectations. There are several chief types of heart conditions:

a. **Arteriosclerosis:** hardening of the arteries, resulting in high blood pressure.
b. **Hypertension:** causes prolonged constriction of vessels and arteries, resulting in high blood pressure.
c. **Rheumatic heart:** caused by an inflammation resulting in damage to or having an adverse effect on muscles and valves.
d. **Congenital heart:** born with heart or imperfect heart, unable to perform correctly.
e. **Mitral stenosis:** hardening or narrowing of valve between left atrium and left ventricle, can be congenital or caused by calcium buildup.

Hardening of the arteries is caused by scar tissue from surgery, infection, or fatty material (cholesterol) lining the artery walls, causing the opening to become smaller. This causes pressure to build, like putting a nozzle on a hose – increasing the force at which it moves in the arteries. The break occurs in the heart or the brain as in a stroke due to this force. Calcium salt deposits along the artery walls in the rough places cause a hardness and the inability of the artery to flex and perform normal peristaltic action. Hardening of the arteries causes several illnesses including heart attacks: normally smooth artery lining becomes rough and narrow because of patchy deposits which interfere with the flow of blood. The rough surface plus the sluggishness of the blood as it moves through too narrow a channel sometimes causes a clot, called Thrombosis. It may block an artery altogether. Sometimes clots break away from the spot where they form and are carried to other parts of the body in the bloodstream. The moving clot is called Embolus. The coronary arteries that nourish the heart muscle itself are more frequently affected by artery hardening than any other. Hardening of these arteries causes a decrease in heart muscle blood supply and may cause the chest pains known as angina pectoris. Coronary thrombosis is the term used when heart attacks occur where a clot forms and occludes or blocks a coronary artery. The aorta is the largest artery. Two coronary arteries supply heart nourishment.

A bowed out, open or closed lesion with only a darker shade than the color of the eye may show on the heart area showing organic heart weakness. A brown spot on the lesion or just a brown spot in the area of the heart shows deterioration of the heart. Deterioration or cardiac damage shows as brown or lesions in an elliptical formation. When there is a splitting separation in the autonomic wreath this shows structural organic weakness of the heart. When there is a pathological disturbance of the aorta, the autonomic nerve wreath seems to separate immediately above the heart area. A thickening of the autonomic nerve wreath at the heart area indicates a tension or spasticity of the heart, neurogenic in origin. If there is an incursion of the autonomic wreath towards the pupil at the heart area, again disturbances in cardiac functions would be of a neurogenic origin. A distention of the colon with an incursion out into the heart area indicates that cardiac disturbances will often result because of gas pockets or impactions in the colon. This causes fibrillation or irregular heart, resulting in eventual heart attacks.

Often there will be no cholesterol showing in the eye and yet the person has a heart attack. In this case it would be of a neurogenic nature, causing a spastic condition of the heart due to overwork, too much stress or nervousness. At this time the autonomic wreath would show this spasticity by an incursion toward the pupil at the heart area of the iris, 14-15 minutes in the left iris.

(4) **CHRONIC COLOR - TOXICITY** See Picture Page 46

After deciding on the texture, focus and heart the next in importance would be the bowel and the autonomic wreath. Death begins in the colon. If we had a clogged up sewer system in our house, we would have more sense than to continue turning on the tap or flushing the toilet, but when it comes to our human sewer system we do not seem to have any conception of its functions. A young medical Doctor writing for a local newspaper, answering an old woman's inquiry regarding constipation, told her it was normal to go as long as five days to a week without a bowel movement. This is the kind of illogical reasoning which is being taught today. When looking in many eyes, it will soon be discovered that most chronic deterioration begins in the bowel and along the autonomic wreath. It will then logically be concluded that the bowel must be kept clean and emptied as often as food is eaten. If you eat 3 meals a day, you should have 3 bowel movements a day. If you eat 3 meals and have one movement, you are becoming constipated not only in the bowels, but in the entire body; waste is backing up in the lymphatic system and having an extreme effect on the brain – a reason for so many headaches and slow thought processes. You will observe that as the body becomes chronically ill, brown splotches or spots begin to appear in the iris of the eye. The iris indicates, as disease progresses, a definite change in the layers of the eye, color wise; for example, the top or main color of the iris is the natural color of a given eye, blue or brown, etc. When we see inherent weakness either in a shadow or a bowed out lesion, the color appears to deepen to a darker shade than the color of the eye. If the body begins to become chronic, the color changes first to a yellow brown, then to darker and darker brown to black, which would be complete deterioration down to the bottom layer of the iris. As the correct diet, vitamins and herbs are followed, the miracle occurs as the iris color changes back from black to brown to light brown to yellow to white to gone. The changes are simultaneously taking place in the body on a continual cleansing basis of good and bad days. When the stage of white is reached often a healing crisis will purge the remaining waste from the body and the eye will clear to its normal color.

(5) **COLON AND STOMACH** See Picture Page 47

The stomach appears on the iris next to the pupil in the first zone. The color appears around the outside of the stomach line with the transverse colon cut in half at the naval, showing half of the transverse colon on the right eye and half on the left eye above the pupil. The ascending colon appears on the right eye paralimbal region adjacent to the stomach area on the ear side of that eye. The small intestines would be then in the center paralimbal region of the stomach area on the nose side of each eye. Wherever the colon or small intestines appear in any other shape than shown on the chart – either an incursion or an excursion with a pocket or sharp points in or out – this indicates a distortion in the colon itself. When there is an incursion toward the pupil, it indicates spasticity, a pinching off of the colon, shrunken in that area. An excursion away from the pupil out of the normal second zone indicates a lack of tone or a distention. Often in this distention there will be brown or black ballooned out pockets deteriorating, showing the colon to be filled with all manner of toxic, chronic waste accumulated possibly for years. This waste clings to the pocket walls of the colon, hardens and fills with worms. If there are pinworms involved, many black dots will appear like black pepper on the color area, if other microscopic parasites are involved, the radii solaris line will seem to project out from the inside of colon line itself. Some radii lines will seem to project from the pupil out like spokes in a wheel, these dark sharp cut lines will often be confused with darkening lesion in the bowel or stomach. In order to change the appearance of a chronic colon on the iris of the eyes, because of changes taking place in the colon itself, it is often necessary to take colonic irrigation along with the mild food diet and cleansing herbs. The herbs psyllium, taken 1-2 tablespoons a day in water or juice, will form a soft bulk attaching itself to the hardened fecal matter in the chronic pockets, pulling off hardened ropelike putrid and rotten waste that has possibly been there for years. Psyllium will then heal the torn places, slippery Elm and okra are also healing and soothing to the sore colon. Goldenseal and cayenne are the herbs that stop internal bleeding; goldenseal is also antibiotic. The cleansing herbs, along with psyllium, a mild food diet and some enemas, can bring the colon back to its normal functions, which is to carry off most of the body waste. Remember, death begins in the colon. Whenever the bowel is chronically ill, vitamin B6 is not produced as it should be to digest and activate our septic tank. The body would be lacking in the natural flora or friendly bacteria. Vitamin B6 added to the diet through acidophilus cultures activates and assists the large and small intestines to accomplish their purposes. Any chronic deterioration on the small intestinal area is a good indication that food is not being properly assimilated. The absorption of nutrients to be used in the body takes place through the small intestinal walls by means of osmosis into the blood stream. If these walls are clogged with tumors, toxic waste, cholesterol or hardened oils, the absorption cannot accurately take place no matter how good the diet may be. When any chronic deterioration shows on the black spotted area shown on the chart as pey-pat (peyers patches), damage could have been done to this area when there was a high fever as a child. Some children did not seem to grow well, and it is found to be for this cause. If the area of the small intestines is only chronically brown or black for other reasons, a cleansing of this part of the body becomes the first and most important step in order to regain health.

Iridology is probably the greatest proof of the effectiveness of a mild food and herb diet. Any time any brown or yellow begins on the iris, this shows that the body is deteriorating in that area. The mild food diet and cleansing herbs are used to clean, changing the picture on the iris. Any good cleansing formula may be used or any of the cancer formulas listed in *Is Any Sick Among You?* It is my opinion that there is only one disease and that is an accumulation of toxic waste in the body. The answer is always the same: clear out the body with herbs and mild food whenever this accumulation begins to show up on the iris of the eyes

(6) **AUTONOMIC WRATH** See Picture Page 47

The autonomic wreath becomes the next in importance when viewing the iris. it is with difficulty that the body will heal when the autonomic wreath is chronic in color. The cleansing of the body becomes very important in order to move the toxic wastes from the nervous system so that other parts will clean more rapidly. If a radio had corrosion on many of the wires, even if you plugged it in and turned it on the radio would not play well. The nervous system is a very intricate and vast system; its messages are carried as secretly as conversation on a telephone wire. Nerve cells look like a drop splashed on a hard surface with tentacles flung out in all directions. The cell body is the central blob, the party sprayed out resembling tree roots are called *dendrites*. Another long single fiber attached is called and *axon;* it ends in a brush like tip. The complete unit is called a neuron. Dendrites except incoming impulses and carry them toward the cell body. The axon carries impulses away from the cell body. Nerves very in diameter according to how many axon fibers are bundled together like cables. Each fiber is an extension of a cell body that may lie a great distance away. The sciatica nerve, for instance, runs from the back to the tip of the toes. Most axons are covered by a white fatty material called myelin. Myelin is like the rubber insulation used on electric wires and may serve other purposes.

Billions of neurons are found in the body – some 12 billion in the brain alone. This is fortunate, for medical science says we cannot regenerate nerve cells. A limited amount of nerve repair is possible as long as the cell body remains intact. The neuron functions in such a way that if a nerve fiber is cut or injured, the part attached to the cell body remains, but the part beyond withers away. Sometimes a live part can extend itself through the withered component to reach its original destination and restore function. In some cases several nerves can be rejoined by a surgeon but only when nerve tracts are accessible; many unfortunately are not.

Electricity follows a continuous wire at a speed of 186,000 miles a second; nerve speed impulses travel only 200 miles an hour. This is fast, but not instantaneous. We cannot safely rely on quick reflexes to get us out of trouble. It takes about 1/10 of a second for nerve impulses to warn us and another split-second to act upon the information, except where extreme fear is involved. In the latter, a shot of adrenaline floods the system. Unfortunately our fear antenna is only geared to certain reflexes by what has been computed into our brain through or by great parental love and training (reaction to a child's cry, etc.).

Nerve impulses travel in a chain reaction, one neuron triggers the next like a train of gunpowder that ignites point by point as heat reaches each neuron. This is an electrochemical process which depends on movements of molecules back and forth across membranes of a nerve fiber. The inside of a resting fiber is negatively charged, the outside positively charged. This is caused by the relative abundance of potassium ions in the interior and sodium ions in the exterior. The firing of a neuron changes the permeability of the membranes with an inward flow of sodium and an outward flow of potassium, reversing the electrical charge. Almost instantly, sodium, potassium movements are reversed and so is the electric charge. These alternating movements of molecules across membranes produce currents that propagate a nerve impulse. Reversals occur as frequently as 1000 times a second; thus, a nerve impulse is a series of tiny electrical breaks which travel over fibers and are boosted from one point to the next by chains of electrochemical relay stations which give local reinforcement of power.

A given stimulus either causes a single neuron to discharge or it does not. Communication between individual neurons is virtually infinite in number since the cells are not physically attached to each other. Such loose connection permits uncountable numbers of switching arrangements. The junction where fine terminal branches of axon come close to dendrites of another neuron, is called synapse. There is no direct contact; the synapse is like a spark gap which a nerve impulse must jump across. The jump is helped by a body chemical, acetylcholine, which is essential for nerve impulse transmission. An excess accumulation compels various organs and tissues to run wild, causing a paralysis like effect (like nerve gas) and a toxic buildup. We have a natural defensive enzyme called cholinesterase which breaks down acetylcholine as fast as it is formed. A fantastically rapid nerve ending buildup and breakdown of opposing chemicals each nerve impulses flowing in good order synapses.

When too much toxic waste is accumulated, the body must operate rapidly to keep up with this, reminding one of an old fashioned movie being run too quickly. When this function becomes worn out and fatigued, what happens then? What happens when certain glands do not function because of the lack of certain hormones or because of overwork, causing fatigue of the glands? What happens when calcium, sodium and potassium balances become imbalanced? There is no difference whatever between nerve impulses except in frequencies per second. There is not a special kind of nerve impulse for seeing and another for smelling or tasting. If some incredibly mischievous rerouting of nerve pathways should occur, we would perhaps be able to hear a flavor or smell a sunset. Something of this nature arises because of glandular imbalance or growths in nervous tissue which may cause unreal but vividly perceived sensations. These are hallucinations of taste, vision and indeed, all senses which have no detectable physical basis. This, in my opinion, is what drugs do (LSD, liquor, etc.). Could it be that drugs settle in spots where nerves cannot function, causing a rerouting or an obstruction in transmission? Could this be how acupuncture works, using an inorganic needle in these places? Since the electrical system works totally on organic substances, could it be that an inorganic substance can clog, or when placed in the correct place, cease transmission?

How important, then, is the autonomic nerve wreath on the iris? In my opinion it is of the utmost importance. This area gives an exact accounting of how far the entire nervous system had deteriorated or is healing. White would show an acute condition, and is interesting to note that when there may be nothing else wrong appearing on the iris and the wreath white, the body can be in a great deal of pain. It naturally follows, then, that cleansing herbs and mild food clean the body of toxic waste accumulated throughout the nervous system. As this is cleansing, other parts will clean also but a complete cleansing of other affected parts of the body does not take place until the wreath is clear. In order to strengthen the nerve activity as it is being cleared, vitamin B complex and calcium of a lactate or gluconate type, along with nervine type herbs, will increase the body's ability to throw off waste.

(7) **NERVE RINGS** See Picture Page 47

Nerve rings appear as a partial or complete line all the way around the iris. The usual white lines indicate that such rings, come and go as there may be inflammation or nerve tension in various parts of the body. A chronic brown color in the rings indicates they have been there a long time. Nerve rings can appear where there is no problem with the autonomic wreath and vice versa. Where the nerve ring crosses the spinal area it can be determined exactly where a chiropractic adjustment will be needed. When the ring follows all the way around the iris in a connected manner the entire body is affected by a nervous condition. When there are 3 rings all the way around, the subject is ready for a nervous breakdown. When there are 4, insanity could one day ensue. There is a more serious condition when rings and wreath are both affected, and paralysis will often appear this way. There will be other things to look for, however. Markings of a chronic spot or lesion on the Medulla in the brain area; markings on the spinal area – paralysis will often appear in this case as a thickening of the autonomic wreath, giving the colon and stomach area a three-dimensional appearance or of being caved in. There will also be markings showing on legs or arm areas if there is a paralysis in either.

It is extremely important to maintain cleanliness of the body tissues in paralysis, especially the bowel as elimination is often slowed down to the point where the body deteriorates very rapidly if this essential process is not taken care of. It is also important to feed the nervous system those elements which soothe and strengthen. Nervine relaxant herbs such as red clover, lobelia, hops, catnip, valerian, chamomile, etc., and the vitamins and minerals necessary to feed the nervous system such as B complex and calcium lactate or calcium gluconate. Of course it is important to remove the cause of stress, if possible. Often a person will not even realize that certain things in his daily life are irritating his nervous system.

(8) **GLANDS** See Picture Page 47

The various glands of the body are in trouble when any marking or lesion appears on the iris of the eyes. The lines of the eyes are normally straight from the autonomic wreath out to the peripheral line of the iris. Wavy lines indicate glandular imbalance. We then look to see which glands are involved. If there are no markings or lesions showing on any of the glands, but the lines are wavy, it is always adrenal imbalance caused from too much stress, a traumatic shock, or a great or extended unsolvable stress.

When the herbs related to various glands are used in a correct balance, the lines will straighten. If there is deterioration in any glands, it is necessary to clean the entire body with mild food and cleansing Herb formulas along with specific hormone herbs. Hormone herbs are as follows:

Pituitary:
Alfalfa – Approximately 10 to 20 or more tablets or capsules.
Adrenal:
Licorice root (acts like natural cortisone) – Approximately 2 to 4 capsules, with mild food. On regular diet and meat, up to 15 capsules.

To get off of cortisone and onto licorice: – Approximately 15 capsules a day until withdrawal is passed – approximately 10 days.

Female:

Black Cohosh (acts like natural estrogen) – Approximately 1 to 3 capsules; if headache, cut back, it is not needed. If a nervous condition persists, another gland is involved. No problem or withdrawal to get off of estrogen and onto black cohosh.

Male:

Ginseng – Approximately 4 to 6 per day no real limit

Sarsaparilla

Pancreas:

Goldenseal root, Juniper (or Cedar berries) (Diabetes) – Approximately 1 to 30 capsules. On a mild food diet, only small amount is necessary, approximately 2 to 4. Juniper berries: approximately 6 to 8 when on mild food.

Hypoglycemia:

Licorice root

Hyperglycemia:

Insulin overshoots its mark, drops to low blood sugar, high and low periods daily or hourly. Will be seen on iris with adrenal as well as pancreas markings. Other glands may be involved, also can eventually become diabetes and Addison's disease. Licorice root, goldenseal root – one half as much as the amount of licorice used.

Adrenals:

When the adrenals are involved, often the thyroid and pituitary and female area also show markings. Eventually becomes Addison's disease. Goldenseal usually not necessary unless sugar is used, causing a pounding heart – steady, consistent low fatigue.

Thyroid:

Will show marking on the thyroid area, lesion or deterioration – check for fluid build-up uric acid, acid stomach and related adrenals.

Hyper, thin type – Kelp, dulse approximately 4 to 6 kelp tablets.

Hypo, fat type – Kelp or dulse liquid approximately 20 drops 70 or more, for fluid buildup on iris field. Potassium gluconate or diuretic herbs to regulate fluids and help thyroid gland in its function. No problem to go off of thyroid drugs onto herbs, no withdrawal; higher doses necessary to regulate,   approximately 20 drops and more, daily.

Dr. E. Hugh Tuckey gave us the valuable information of hydrochloric acid (Footnote as Found in National Health Federation Bulletin October 1967) for use in digestion. He said that the major role of hydrochloric acid is to digest protein and if there is too little hydrochloric acid, the stomach does not empty as soon as usual and foods eaten 3 to 4 days earlier, not digested causes putrefaction, gas, a belching condition, and a burning in the stomach, a substernal burning just behind the breastbone. He says further that a person with these problems will then take a bicarbonate of soda or other type of antacid to alkalize a stomach that already does not have enough acid, when often the antacid used will be an aluminum preparation which he says can cause cancer.

He states also that on tests, lactic acid shows up in the stomach in these cases and it does not belong there at all. When the emptying time of the stomach is slowed down due to hypo- or anachlorhydria, he says we always find a spastic pylorus and we can demonstrate this clinically one hundred times out of a hundred; we don't have to guess at it. Then he has shown how the spasticity in turn involves the bile duct and pancreatic duct. If the pylorus is in a state of spasm, the duodenum is also in a state of spasm so a normal amount of bile is not emptying into the small intestines. One of the properties of bile is a bactericide along with promoting the peristalsis of the small intestines. This also causes the liver to become engorged with bile that should be going to the small intestines. The pancreas is also affected, causing a backing up of its secreting substances and the pancreas them becomes enlarged, hard and extremely tender. We can see that this lack of hydrochloric acid has far-reaching effects involving the stomach, liver, gallbladder, pancreas, assimilation of food, constipation and pancreatitis and even hepatitis. Doctor Tuckey gave hydrochloric acid to his patients so that people could handle the protein and found that they would have to take these on an indefinite basis unless they were given a pancreatic, duodenal substance, then the hydrochloric acid would normalize in 2 to 4 months. Doctor

Tuckey was not clear on the cause of the problem but rather thought it could be caused from emotions and the stress of everyday incompatible living conditions. He has given us some very valuable information resulting from 30 years of research. He mentions also the use of hydrochloric acid tablets when traveling in countries where there is bad water, for killing the amoebas in the water and preventing diarrhea discomfort while traveling. It is with apprehension that I mentioned his findings and I wish to add rather than distract from his work. It has been by discovery that the cause is as he had supposed an adrenal cortial exhaustion causing a lack of the adrenal cortin hormone which interferes with the production of hydrochloric acid, causing a uric acid buildup in the stomach. This is also the cause of the lactic acid build he mentioned resulting from any exercise. The lactic acid builds in the muscles from exercise and the excess is normally routed back to the liver and changed to glycogen and used again as energy. This seepage through the of abdominal wall could result because the liver is too badly clogged in the way he has described and so seeps into the abdominal tissue and into the stomach, causing the burning sensations experienced when lactic acid is present in the stomach.

The experience I have had shows me that licorice root acts like the adrenal hormone relieving the mental stress but this hydrochloric problem is relieved by saffron, to open the clogged liver, having a definite effect on oil, and assist the pancreatic functions and then dandelion dispels the uric acid which has built up in the stomach and the rest of the body – somehow regulating the hydrochloric as a natural magnesium or anti-acid effect on the body, without the side effects of taking an anti-acid such as soda.

(9) **OPEN LESIONS** See Picture Page 47- 48

Open lesions are inherent weaknesses when they are just a color shade darker than the color of the iris. Any darkening shades down into lower layers indicate chronic deterioration in varying stages. Open lesions heal faster than closed lesions. Lesions that are chronic will sometimes net, having the appearance of a darned sock. Lines will weave closer and closer at times closing the lesion when corrective measures in diet and herbs are taken; other times they may clean to a color shade darker than the eye and remain. Chronic deterioration begins usually on the outside edge of the lesion moving from outside to center in varying stages of chronic color from yellow to brown to black but as it begins to heal, white will appear on the top and around edges with the knitting appearance. Colors underneath gradually lighten and colors on top become whiter and whiter until they disappear.

(10) **CLOSED LESIONS** See Picture Page 48

A closed lesion is more serious than an open lesion and is more difficult to heal. When white knitting lines begin to appear it is a good indication that the problem can be solved, otherwise the same would apply to the closed lesion as with the open lesion.

(11) **PARASITES** See Picture Page 48

Parasites are often the reason people who have fasted off and on for years and lived on a good diet never quite reach the stage of good health they work so hard for. Parasites live on the refuse of the body hold onto the waste even in a fasting state – especially in a fasting state, as it is their food supply. The only time they turn loose of it is when they are killed; then the mucus in which they live sloughs off like a healing crisis.

The radii solaris spokes which look like a dark, sharp cut line on the iris indicate heavy parasite involvement in the particular part of the body where they are showing. When the parasites are killed, the lines begin to flatten and fuzz off; then disappear altogether. The so-called radiation lines which are wider than radii solaris spokes are also involved with parasites of a stronger variety. Pumpkin seed and herbal pumpkin formulas will usually take care of radii solaris spokes but it takes Black Walnut to change the radiation lines. The time it takes to get rid of them varies depending on how deeply entrenched they are. A crisis can occur when mucus sloughs off and lasts anytime from 2 weeks to 6 or 8 months. Sometimes no real crisis is necessary for the mucus just begins to move a little at a time. As parasites are killed, a smelly drainage is caused if it is near a body opening such as in the head area, kidney, vagina or rectum.

Parasites were a definite pathological concept in ancient Egyptian medicine as shown by the graphic reproduction of animals in mural paintings, comprising an important part of certain hieroglyphics that indicate disease. In Egyptian pathology the animal was considered the symbol of disease. Ra, the sun God, falls sick because of a worm born from his sputum, when the parasite is not visible, an invisible worm is imagined.

During the period when Egypt passed under domination of Persia, the decay in medicine began. The conquerors tried to preserve ancient traditions in medicine but the physician was so closely attached to the religious priests and government rule, as this changed hands the brilliant medical practices decayed into sorcery and charlatan drug vendors, similar to what has happened in the past 50 years to our society. Our grandmothers were well acquainted with de-worming their children, but today we only de-worm our dogs.

(12) **INJURY**

Injury will show up in many shapes and forms with all lines irregularly crossing natural lines. Toxic waste a deterioration follows the regular line pattern of the iris from pupil to peripheral line but an injury can cross in all or any direction, this is what makes it easily discernible.

(13) **SURGERY**

A surgery will look at times as though a hole was cut out of the iris in all shapes and sizes. A broken bone will usually show a straight cut line crossing the bone area where the break occurred. An injury or a surgery may, if permanent damage is done, turn a brown color and remain that way even though a cleansing diet and herbs are extensively used.

(14) **DRUGS** See Picture Page 48

Drugs can be easily identified on the iris of the eye by a sodium ring which is a gray-white or brown ring around a peripheral line on the 6th and 7th zones. This ring appears to be super-imposed above

34

the top layer. Drugs are also revealed as a red or bright brown circle around the outside edge of the pupil.

What is meant by the word "drug"? In centuries past, the word "drug" was used synonymously with herbs or medicine. As herbs became obsolete to the medical world and were replaced by chemical drugs, herbs were no longer classed as drugs. Some drugs of a chemical nature are made by mixing chemicals with herbs. In this case the herb is still classed as a drug because of the chemical additive. The chemicals used to make drugs are inorganic substances, such as potash, salts or petroleum. We then have another drug factor used which is made from organic narcotic herbs, such as morphine, caffeine, nicotine, etc. Some are used in the natural state, many others are used in conjunction again with chemical salts or potash. In order to identify those botanicals classed as drugs, we find that all must be named with a name ending in "ine" whether in a natural state or as a mixture with other salt chemicals.

Hard narcotic drugs show up on the pupil red ring and whenever brown spots appear to be super-imposed over the top layer of the iris. Furthermore, drugs of a narcotic or a salt nature both have an effect on the autonomic wreath and when it appears to be chronic in color. Drugs are inhibiting the normal routing of the nerve signals through the area of the body where such chronic color appears on the wreath. Sometimes the entire wreath will appear chronic in color: this is another reason for a cleanse to rid the body of the inorganic drug substances interfering with nerve impulses. This is also the reason for the side effects of drugs. When the nervous system is malfunctioning it is with difficulty that the body heals. As drastic changes in the iris occur because of the chemical salts of drugs, the dangers of drugs become more apparent. All of these markings of the brown chronic nature, whether drug caused or incorrect eating habits and poor nutrition, are indicative of deteriorating disease. It makes no difference what the cause, when we see the shadows of doom registering the extent of deterioration in the body, it is time to find out what we have been doing wrong and make a change for the better.

(15) **ACUTE CONDITION** See Picture Page 48

An acute condition in the body is shown on the iris as white over the top of the main color layer. The condition such as a cold, flu, measles, mumps, chickenpox, etc., will all show white over most of the iris field. There are varying degrees of white: the more heavily the body is eliminating, the whiter the eyes become, as the elimination passes out of the body, the white will gradually disappear. Some people have white on the eyes all the time. This type of person has a good ability to eliminate and is in a constant state of elimination they are always fatigued and weak, the way one feels when he has a cold without the fever. This type of individual would do well rapidly and remain well if he would stop the intake of concentrated or poor foods which the body is always trying to throw off.

Often when the body is chronically sick and an attempt is made to fast, or semi-fast by mild food diet and herbs, the body will begin to eliminate and the eyes will whiten as the elimination begins to take place. "Acute" means toxic waste on the move in the blood stream on its way out. White always means healing, whether nature's forcing an elimination as with a cold to save life, or whether an elimination is caused by a semi-fast, etc.

In case of an inflammation, white would show in the inflamed area as white on the top of the top color layer. White appearing deeply in between the lines indicates parasites coupled with an acute pain such as would be caused in lupus, rheumatoid arthritis, or malaria. The white line may turn dark and become a radius solaris showing only that the parasites are more deeply entrenched and of a chronic nature. Because white is always of an acute nature, pain is always involved where white is showing. In the case where parasites are involved, the body can remain in an acute, painful condition as the toxic waste just stirs around in the blood stream and is unable to leave the body. In these cases the parasites must be killed in order to eliminate the waste. As healing begins to occur, white lines will appear around the spot or crisscrossing white lines where chronic disease is involved. Sometimes healing looks like someone placed a white screen across the Brown spots leaving the Brown showing underneath.

(16) **LIVER, GALL BLADDER** see Picture Page 48

36

Any chronic deterioration showing on the liver and gallbladder causes a difficulty with healing. Sometimes the bowel is blocked causing the liver to malfunction. The bowel area must be checked to see if it shows a toxic condition. If so, this would be the first thing to clear out in order for the liver to empty and clean. When chronic color shows in the gallbladder, gallstones could be the problem. The gallbladder purge as related in *Is Any Sick Among You?* could be used to empty the gallbladder stones so that normal elimination can be carried on. The other place to look in conjunction with the liver and gallbladder would be the duodenum. If there is an ulceration showing or a chronic color, slippery elm is the herb soothing to ulceration.

(17) **KIDNEYS** See Picture Page 49

The kidneys are a very important part of the body's ability to eliminate. We have 4 main organs of elimination: bowel, kidneys, lungs and skin. When any of these is clogged or malfunctioning, it places an added burden on the others. It is therefore important to keep each one of these organs functioning well. If there is a chronic condition appearing on the iris either in a lesion or a spot, special care must be taken to make sure the bowel is free and clear. If there is an acute condition – white showing on the kidney area – the bowel must be kept almost loose in order the damage will not be done to the body. When a person has a fairly strong eliminative ability at the onset of an acute kidney infection, the bowels will automatically become loose in order to save the kidneys and reroute the fluids through the bowel. Lemons and vitamin C help to dissolve the mucous and any stones. Goldenseal is an antibiotic for any germs, while kidney herbs listed on the chart are for restoration. When the inflammation appears a gray, metallic color, and over acidic condition exists. Dandelion and saffron, fill and vitamin C dispel acids.

(18) **BONES** See Picture Page 49

On the iris chart the bony areas are well-defined: shoulder, scapula, thoracic (rib cage), spinal, leg (thigh, knee and foot), hand and arm, pelvis, and the neck are represented (the latter on the medulla). The top of the head appears at 12 o'clock; back of the head towards 1 o'clock; jaw, nose, face and skin area close to the periphery. A break will cross the normal lines of the iris and can show if the bone has been shattered or a clean break. When deterioration has set in, the break will show as brown or black – otherwise crisscross, jagged, odd shaped markings depending upon the break itself.

Often in an old break, even one that was well set, arthritis will set in and will also appear to be brown in color. If it is a damaged deterioration of bone and surrounding tissue, the brown color may never change. If it is an arthritic condition, irreversible changes may occur in bone shape but the brown showing deterioration may leave the iris. The brown or black – if it is arthritis in the bone – will show on the 6th zone on the bony area.

Hypercalcemia will appear as a gray-white color. If it is general in the whole body, the entire iris color will appear to be gray-white. When it is specifically causing sight problems, a gray glandular appearance will appear on either side of the pupil. A calcium problem in the body, whether it is settling in the arteries, in the joints, or in the tissues, involves the adrenal and parathyroid glands.

In order to regulate the correct calcium metabolism, glands need to be properly functioning and secreting their necessary hormones. When they are unable to perform accurately, either because of too much stress or organic weakness, many things begin to malfunction. The bowel begins to ulcerate, and the kidneys are then overworked and malfunction, causing fluid to build up in the tissues. The skin backs up trying to carry off waste and causes a splotchy pigmentation. The liver does not function as it should, breaks or lesions begin to occur in the inner abdominal wall, allowing a seepage of lactic acid into the stomach and interfering with digestion. Lactic acid is not changed to glycogen by the liver so as to be used again as energy and a toxic condition begins to increase. The result is complete fatigue, exhaustion, mental problems and nervousness.

Fluid buildup in the body and around the heart and eyes causes sight problems and heart weakness with a possible uric acid buildup or burning sensation. It can be determined just how far hypercalcemia has gone by checking each of these organs mentioned. In order to

38

bring the calcium back to normal ossification when the body is not producing adequate hormones, the herbal hormone type herbs will sustain life the way insulin does in a diabetic. Where there is an extreme uric acid and lactic acid buildup, saffron and dandelion are helpful herbs. The adrenal hormone type herb is licorice; the parathyroid hormone type herbs are alfalfa and kelp.

Osteoporosis is a calcium lack where insufficient calcium is taken into the body and the body begins (activated by the parathyroid glands) to leach calcium from the bones in order to maintain correct calcium levels in the blood. The bones then become hollow and brittle. This often happens with old people who live on bland diets not rich in calcium and other minerals. This is a cause of much of the senility in old age, because in order for the brain to function, blood calcium must be kept at correct levels. Even in a hypercalcemia condition where calcium is deposited in the body, the person could have too low a level of calcium in the blood. This is the cause of the mental breakdown common to the hypo and hyperglycemia type. Whenever an arc or crescent appears across the upper portion of the iris brain area – looking as if the white were pulled down over the upper iris obscuring the peripheral line – it is an indication of senility beginning because of the lack of calcium to the brain. By helping the glands and the calcium metabolize in the body, senility can often be thwarted. Sometimes, however, the arc is caused by brain damage, and senility is the result anyway. An osteoporosis or hollowing out of the bone condition appears on the body structures of the body in the iris as a pit-like appearance, like cement that has not been troweled enough. The addition of calcium and related mineral which cause calcium to be utilized in the body will readily regulate this condition.

(19) EYES

The eye section of the iris would show no markings unless there were inherent weakness shadow lines or lesions. When a dark discoloration begins to appear, deterioration is beginning to occur to eyesight. Related organs that can cause site problems need to be checked: kidneys, glands, bowels and nerve wreath. In order to help the sight, all related organs must be helped also. An infection in the eyes or hay fever, etc., will show a white line on top of the top color layer.

(20) **EARS** See Picture Page 49

With the ear, it would be the same as with the eyes. Sometimes, however, parasites may have invaded the glands around the ear and neck to the extent that a radiation line will appear on the iris. This radiation line – or parasites – will cause eventual prostration of the nerves and can cause nerve deafness. Watch for radii Solaris lines and radiation on eye area also.

(21) **ANEMIA** See Picture Page 49

Anemia is a word not correctly understood. Unless there has been hemorrhaging, the need for iron is a very small amount. This arc is often accompanied with a scurf rim, placing an added burden on the internal skin and other organs of elimination. This should indicate that toxic waste is accumulating in the area of the arc, and has difficulty in moving itself out. Anemia means an encumbrance of toxic waste in the blood. It is interesting to note that when the white blood count is high and the system is cleansed with herbs and mild food, the white count goes down and the red count goes up. When the system is cleaned, the arc clears off the iris.

(22) **SCURF RIM** Picture Page 49

The scurf rim suggests condition of the skin. Anytime the peripheral line is wider than a pencil line this is called a scurf rim, and it may widen as far as the fifth zone. The uniformity of depths can very all around the circumference of the iris, indicating that the skin may be better in one place than another. The darker and more defined the color and the wider the ring, the greater the impairment of skin function and the retention of toxic waste. If the color is only a shade darker than the color of the iris and a scurf rim is showing to any extent, this is only inherent weakness. Other problems will result if the bowel and kidneys cannot carry off the waste properly. The skin is the third kidney, and when it is not functioning well, the entire body suffers. Wherever there is an incursion of the scurf rim, the area of incursion becomes more readily toxic in that part of the body. When the lymphatic rosary nodule appears to have spilled over into the scurf rim showing a white line, this indicates swelling or fluid buildup in the tissues of that area of the body, revealing these white lines on the iris.

(23) **LYMPHATIC ROSARY** See Picture Page 50

The lymphatic rosary on the iris often looks like globs or nodules of white, yellow or brown beads strung around the sixth zone. Sometimes they connect all the way around. Other times they are disconnected and show only sparsely around the circumference of the sixth zone. Any time these globs show on the iris anywhere on this zone, it is an indication of an accumulation of mucus waste in the lymph of the body. If the color is extremely white – almost blue – it appears to be superimposed on the top of the fibers of the iris, it is considered as an index of arsenic retention in the lymph system. Whether the lymphatic rosary appears white, yellow, or brown and to have a thickening of the fibers themselves, this would indicate lymph congestion only. Often there is arsenic retention as well as mucus congestion of the lymph, making it difficult to distinguish. The arsenic retained in the lymph is related to neuritis conditions and will become neuritis later as it becomes more chronic. This is also related to arthritis.

There are seven zones from pupil to peripheral line. The sixth zone where the lymphatic rosary is found, has also to do with circulation. When circulation is poor, the lymph nodes and the body began to retain waste. As waste is retained in the lymph, the thyroid works overtime to send iodine into the body to kill the germs living in the mucus waste accumulating. When thyroid activity is increased, pituitary activity is decreased, as they act like a balance scale: increase of one decreases the other. When thyroid activity is increased, oxidation increases to assist the body in expelling waste the same way we breathe faster when we have a cold or flu. The spleen is also overworked since it acts like the vacuum system of the body, and it is then overworked causing a breakdown in its ability to do its job accurately – a lowering of resistance to infection. This is not a valid assumption, however, because all that has to be done is clean the body of toxic waste, and normal function will be resumed.

There are a few other places necessary to know not listed on the chart which occur in rarer cases. Wilson's disease causes a copper colored ring to appear on the seventh zone or skin area. Multiple sclerosis shows markings of deterioration on the medulla and spine. The autonomic wreath and colon will appear very toxic. When paralysis has begun, markings on the arm and leg areas appear on the iris and the autonomic wreath will usually separate at the medulla area. If calcification has begun, the iris color changes to a gray-white and the autonomic wreath appears to be raised, while the colon appears to be sunken in. Calcification can change the pressure of cerebrospinal fluid and have an effect on the choroid plexus which regulates these fluids. Other times gland malfunctions can have an effect on this fluid, which affects the spine and brain.

If the pressure of the cerebrospinal fluid is not kept stable, the entire body can be affected. Many pathological and functional disturbances then begin to occur: digestive, respiratory, headache, circulatory ailments causing general slowing down of eliminative processes which result in a general toxic condition. When this happens, legs can be affected – anything from varicose veins to paralysis of legs and feet and could even begin with a gouty condition. When other glands are not functioning properly (especially the adrenal glands) the cerebrospinal fluid pressure can be lowered, resulting in the above pathological disturbances. In either case, calcification or cerebrospinal lowering or pressure are the result of glandular imbalance which will also appear as wavy lines on the iris.

When individual or collective gland problems are solved by hormone herbs and corrective diet, the calcification is halted and normal ossification begins again. Since the choroid plexus is a gland also secreting hormones, alfalfa is the regulatory natural hormone herbs for the choroid plexus. An acid stomach will appear as a gray color on stomach area, but here again normal ossification is beginning to be disturbed, it is caused by certain gland imbalances of the body – deterioration in the medulla or other glands or merely an intolerable stress which throws the glands out of balance.

The medulla may be observed for many malfunctions: that the glands affect the medulla or did the medulla cause the glandular imbalance? Parasites should be watched for in the medulla or any other deterioration or inflammation. The medulla can have far-reaching effects on the body since it regulates saliva, controls respiration, controls cerebrospinal fluids, swallowing, heart, vomiting, sneezing, and sweating. Whenever deterioration shows on the medulla, any of the above symptoms or pathological problems can be the result, making it doubly important to use cleansing herbs. Certain asthma cases and even multiple sclerosis could be caused by a defect in the medulla. Twitching of the muscles is usually a lack of magnesium, but where magnesium does not stop the twitching eye or muscles, it is then caused by the lack of the parathyroid hormones calcitonin or parathormone. Here again alfalfa is the answer, regulating the parathyroid's in their function. As with other brown deterioration markings showing on the ris, cleansing herbs and regulatory hormones along with mild food are the solutions to the problem.

Let me say again there is only one disease and that is an accumulation of toxic waste. This accumulation happens because of incorrect eating habits, improper nutrition or inherent weakness. When there is inherent organic weakness, a better nutrition and more care must be taken to live a better, healthier life. When the body is filled to the limit with toxic waste mucus, the only way to better health is to clean it out. The only way to clean it out is to stop the intake of concentrated, mucus forming foods so that mucus waste can eliminate from the body. Herbs are a great help in this elimination process, causing the mucus to dissolve and eliminate more rapidly. Some herbs are meant to kill the bacteria and parasites living on the mucus so that the mucus they hold onto and live in to survive can be released and expelled. Many herbs can be taken together, working like a fine team – a precision machine to cleanse, soothe and heal, each one having an almost innate intelligence which directs it to the special place in the body where it functions. The greatest secret to good health is to keep the body clean inside as well as out.

Many important and knowledgeable people are coming to the conclusions that we have far too long heralded the virtues of meat protein even to the exclusion of the use of necessary mineral foods.

In an article from *Today's Health,* Daniel Grotta Kurska points out that scientists have long classified meat as first-class protein and vegetables as second-class, thereby implying that non-animal protein is somehow inferior. Current evidence, however, points to other conclusions.

The steps to the top of the ladder of disease are as follows, as we start up the tree of disease:

TREE OF DISEASE

7. Symptom level (pain)
6. Parasite and germ infiltration
5. Increased oxidation
4. Decreased pituitary activity
3. Increased thyroid activity
2. Lymphatic retention
1. Normal body chemical balance

PICTORAL SECTION

The following pages of eye photographs have tried to illustrate the various problems found in selected Iris. Pictures have been enlarged making it easier for the naked eye to detect the problems. The pictures from pages 51 to 55 relate to chapter 2 of this book. The pictures on the remaining pages are our "Before and After" group. These are the Iris of some brave souls that have discovered their problems and are striving to correct them.

Reference is made here to pictures in the "Before and After quote group that have corresponding testimonies in the body of the book:

Gary Gillum – testimony page 163; bottom two pictures page 53

Wyonna Kruse – testimony page 173; top four pictures page 53

Jeannine McKenzie – testimony page 167; three pictures page 54, left section

Ruth Ruhland – testimony page 80; two pictures page 56 right section

Michael Tracy – testimony page 167; top two pictures page 52

No. 1 TEXTURE
See page 20

No. 2 FOCUS LINES
See page 20

No. 3a HEART
See page 20

No. 3b HEART
See page 20

No. 4a CHRONIC
COLOR - TOXICITY
See page 22

No. 4b CHRONIC
COLOR - TOXICITY
See page 22

No. 5a COLON &
STOMACH
See Page 23

No. 5b COLON &
STOMACH
See Page 23

No. 6 AUTONOMIC
WREATH
See Page 25

No. 7 NERVE RINGS
See Page 28

No. 8 GLANDS
See page 29

No. 9 OPEN LESIONS
See Page 32

No. 9 OPEN LESIONS
LESIONS
See Page 32

No. 10 CLOSED

See Page 33

No. 11 PARASITES
14 DRUGS
See page 33

No.

See Page 34

No. 15 ACUTE
        No. 16 LIVER -   CONDITION
                    GALLBLADDER
    See Page 35

No. 17 KIDNEYS
    No. 18 BONES
  See Page 37
    See Page 37

No. 20 EARS
    No. 21A ANEMIA
  See Page 39
    See Page 40

No. 21B ANEMIA
    No. 22 SCURF RIM
  See Page 40
      See Page 40

No. 23 LYMPHATIC ROSARY
See Page 41

Adult female – maintains good diet – flat focus; week vitality; some spots; yellow color; mucus in entire body

One month later – after heavy elimination from taking high doses of herbal formula color changes to

blue; her focus; much improvement

Adult female – good texture but many spots dark brown to lower layers of deterioration

2 years later using mild food diet and herbs, passed much mucus; spots lighter and smaller; general

color improvement; still a ways to

Adult female – chronic bowel and stomach; lymphatic rosary; weak glands; prolapsed colon; shadow weakness

18 months later, not much diet change but used many herbs – lymphatic rosary whitening; shadows

lightening; note area 3:00 almost

Adult male – young; parasites;   *Stayed on mild food and herbs for*
chronic overall condition serious   *6 months and the color is beginning*

to change; spots going; parasites

going

Adult female – chronic bowel;   *Note   drastic   changes*
after few
autonomic wreath; spots; parasites;   *months mild food diet and herbs*
bowel darkened to lower layer

Was told by Doctor she had terminal   *Note drastic changes after few*
cancer – a year to live   *months mild food diet*
and herbs

Serious bowel; chronic bowel and autonomic wreath; chronic mucus in entire body; spots in colon parasites

Some improvement in a few months on mild food diet and herbs waste begins to gather to colon

area as outer areas of the body

eliminate and

5 months later very white on chronic in improved color area lightening; gone; parasite lines heavy elimination; spots going

Color improvement; still bowel; spots almost gone

Adult male – serious over-all diet chronic condition; parasites; entire weakness; flat focus

After several years of mild food and herbs – parasite lines show better as other waste is eliminated;

sharper focus; increased vitality;

Adult –2nd picture after several months of mild food diet & herbs; beginning to whiten as elimination proceeds; lesions dark into lower layers; shadow weakness areas down to lower layers; heavy deterioration; chronic autonomic wreath; shrunken bowel; Brown spot; scurf rim

Child – dark lesions into lower layers; infection; lymphatic rosary; bowel spastic descending colon; acid stomach; some spots; scurf rim; chronic bowel

8 months later lesions lightened; eyes whitened; color improved; autonomic wreath improved; scurf rim smaller; nerve ring improved

8 months later – mild food diet with some herbs – all lesions lightening; improved scurf rim; chronic bowel improved

months later – all lesions shadow weakness lighter; color brighter; scurf rim improved; heavy nerve ring almost gone; spots gone

4 months later – brighter color; bowel improved to almost normal; lesions lightened and smaller scurf rim much improved

Child with serious shattered appearance and lesions down to lower layers; spastic colon; scurf rim; heavy nerve ring

Child – fair texture; some shadow of inherent weakness; chronic color; acid stomach; parasites in head area; scurf rim wide; chronic and acute mucus around autonomic wreath

Mild food diet for eight months with some herbs; eye whitening; smaller scurf rim; lesions lightening

8 months on mild food diet with some herbs – colon improved; acid stomach gone; eyes whitening; heavy elimination

4 months later – smaller scurf rim; lighter lesions; nerve ring gone; more blue color; eyes still white; elimination continuing with improved colon line

4 months later – color more blue; still eliminating; parasites gone; scurf rim much smaller

Child with inherent lesions; darkened down into lower layers – serious

Refer to testimony – prior to this photo tumor of the bowel was passed; tumor also from female area; chronic bowel; autonomic wreath; chronic mucus entire body

Mild food diet except school lunch – 6 months with very little herb's – eye's begin to whiten; lesions lightening

After healing crisis color changes in eye from brown to blue; still some work to do

1 year – continued mild food diet with the exception of school lunch; some herbs – lesions lightening; color blue more pronounced; spots fading

Colon spots; chronic autonomic wreath; dark inherent weakness shadows; chronic mucus in blood is yellow cast; parasite lines;

After a few months, not much diet change, more blue showing and lighter; shadow colon spots diminishing; parasite lines fading to white healing lines

The above patient, José, has been a patient 15 years, at the Santa Maria De Tequepexpan Leprosario, Guadalajara, Mexico. This was the day we started treatments, amid the doubts of the doctor and Padre, but we had God on our side and it worked!

Eight weeks later, a vast amount of improvement. The foot is no longer withered, and the calf, after 15 years of disintegration seems to be forming near-normal. The new, pink healthy flesh, is converging from both sides and the top, on the disappearing lesion. In another 8 to 10 weeks, the patient will be dismissed and permitted to go home.

IRIDOLOGY CHART

1. Texture:

Excellent	Good	Fair	Poor
Fine not chronic.	Some lesions, darkening	Lesion darkened	Shattered, lesions

For Desired Change: if inherently poor texture usually not possible to make a change but must live a more healthy life than those having a finer texture, in order to survive and remain well.

2. Focus Lines:

Excellent	Good	Fair	Poor
Sharp	Medium sharp	Flat	Out of focus

For Desired Change: can be changed in many cases by eating more live, especially in old age. When the old go to a softer diet and fewer raw foods, dark chronic color is increased. When many raw juices are added to their diet, the strength will increase and focus will sharpen where focus is already flat, showing weakness. More food and vitamins will sharpen the focus increasing endurance and strength.

3. Heart:

Excellent	Good	Fair	Poor
No lesions or markings of any kind.	No wreath involvement No lesions, excursion of autonomic wreath into heart area. Would still be all right. Must be corrected.	Inherent lesions, no spots, involvement of autonomic wreath.	Lesions and spots or involvement of autonomic wreath.

For Desired Change: Usually cleaning colon and entire body relieves the burden on the heart, but too much toxic waste moving too fast pumping through the heart as the body expels, can cause more damage, like taking a shot of deadly poison. People with heart problems must move slowly, eliminating with mild food and cleansing herbs and must not try to fast or go on fruit only. Herbs that cancel out poison, such as saffron and dandelion, should be used. Then heart herbs such as Hawthorn (strengthen and rejuvenate the heart), potassium gluconate (strengthen the heart muscle) and vitamin E may be taken. One of the most deadly poisons to hurt the heart in the process of elimination is uric acid. We're kidneys are not properly carrying off the waste, dandelion and saffron have a way of neutralizing this uric acid. Other kidney herbs help to activate the kidneys to a better function. Potassium gluconate and celery juice also help to pull off fluid. Where the kidneys will not respond to such methods, the bowel must be forced to evacuate to a fluid state by highly laxative herbs. This takes the burden temporarily off of the kidneys and causes waste to flush out rather than circulate through the heart.

4. Chronic Color-toxicity, spots or shaded:

Excellent	Good	Fair	Poor
Natural color of eye.	Beginning to color into yellow or	Brown spots, light brown in lesions. light brown.	Lesions deteriorating to lower layer black.

For Desired Change: Any chronic spots or lesions showing deterioration, mild food and cleansing herbs until spots are removed and healing is complete. Often people feel better; so stop and go back to concentrated foods before they have sufficiently cleansed.

5. Colon and Stomach:

Excellent	Good	Fair	Poor
Normal colon stomach lines outlined only by darker shades than eye color.	Some deterioration, no chronic color.	Distention of incursion to pupil, darkening spots or lesions	Distention or incursions to pupil, dark spots or lesions or parasites.

For Desired Change: Enemas, cleansing herbs, mild food diet, parasite herbs, psyllium, slippery elm (for ulceration or soreness, fissures or hemorrhoids). Cayenne and goldenseal for any bleeding vitamin B₆ or acidophilus.

6. Autonomic Wreath:

Excellent	Good	Fair	Poor
Outlining only darker shade than color of the eye. Medium thickness all the way around.	Good thickness, white or light brown in color.	Uneven thickness, darkening in color.	Uneven thickness or very thin, darkening color, splitting separations.

For Desired Change: Nervine herbs (see *Is Any Sick Among You?),* Vitamin B complex, calcium lactate or gluconate, cleansing herbs, mild food.

7. Nerve Rings:

Excellent	Good	Fair	Poor
No rings showing.	Small and few showing.	One or two disconnected rings, white in color.	Brown rings two or more, three or more white rings

For Desired Change: Where chronic showing, check nerve wreath also. When white nerve rings come and go, find out who or what is causing a nervous tension. Change environment or attitude towards environment. B complex, calcium lactate or gluconate and nervine herbs.

8. Glands:

Excellent	Good	Fair	Poor
No marks or lesions on gland areas, straight lines	Possible wavy lines but no markings or lesions on	Lesions on glands, no deterioration, wavy lines.	Lesions, wavy lines, deterioration or spots

on iris.　　　　gland area.　　　　　　　　appearing on
　　　　　　　　　　　　　　　　　　　　gland areas.

For Desired Change: Mild food diet and cleansing herbs. Add herbs specific to the gland effected. (see *Is Any Sick Among You?)*

9. Open Lesions; extent of deterioration, determine which organ:

Excellent	Good	Fair	Poor
None showing.	Small lesions only a shade darker than iris.	Few larger lesions with some deterioration showing.	Many lesions, much deterioration, brown and black.

For Desired Change: Open lesions are easier to change because waste has a way out. Mild foods and cleansing herbs.

10. Closed Lesions; extent of deterioration, determine which organ:

Excellent	Good	Fair	Poor
None showing.	Small lesions only a shade darker than iris.	Few larger lesions with some deterioration showing.	Many lesions, much deterioration, brown and black.

For Desired Change: Same as above but more difficult to change. Healing lines will appear across lesions as if you were weaving crisscross threads over the lesions.

11. Parasites:

Excellent	Good	Fair	Poor
No chronic deterioration, no radii solaris lines or radiation lines.	Any chronic disease, radii solaris lines.	Any chronic disease, radii solaris lines, radiation lines.	Heavy showing of chronic disease, radii solaris lines radiation lines especially on animation area.

For Desired Change: Where cancer parasites (progenitor cryptocide) cancer formulas, sometimes additional herbs such as chaparral and black Walnut. Where Salmonella and trichinosis: pumpkin seed (also see herbal pumpkin formula in *Is Any Sick Among You?*). Where Lupus, malaria or leprosy: black Walnut. Lines will fuzz off then go to white, then disappear as parasites are killed.

12. Injury

Excellent	Good	Fair	Poor
No injury	Injury from infection adhesions.	Some, of a minor nature.	Brain damage from stroke or other heavy injury.

For Desired Change: For injury causing scar tissue, vitamin E. Must live on a better-than-average diet, depending on damage done.

13. Surgery:

Excellent	Good	Fair	Poor
No surgery	Minor surgery	Scar tissue, adhesions, minor surgery brown or black.	Major surgery black & brown spot remaining even after cleansing diet.

For Desired Change: Scar tissue, same as above. When permanent damage has been done, area will remain Brown or black.

14. Drugs:

Excellent	Good	Fair	Poor
No drugs showing.	Some small sodium rings in one area.	Sodium ring medium.	Large sodium ring and drug red ring around pupil.

For Desired Change: Drugs can be expelled as the body is placed in a fasting or semi-fasting state. As they move into circulation, palpitations will often occur. Care must be taken in the elimination process when many drugs have been taken of an extremely toxic nature. Taking care of the heart as has been mentioned, mild foods and cleansing herbs. (See heart)

15. Acute:

Excellent	Good	Fair	Poor
No white showing.	Small amount of white showing.	When eliminating, large amounts of white showing.	When NOT eliminating and large amounts of white showing.

For Desired Change: Acute inflammation or acute illness when eyes show white over the top of the iris color, waste is on the move in the blood, help nature get the waste out of the body. Fruit only, cleansing herbs, laxative herbs, high doses of vitamin C and enemas.

16. Liver, Gall Bladder:

Excellent	Good	Fair	Poor
No markings showing.	Shadow darker than iris color indicating weakness.	Either liver or gallbladder, showing chronic color.	Both liver and gallbladder shows chronic color.

For Desired Change: Mild food and cleansing herbal formula. Gallbladder purge (see *Is Any Sick Among You?*). Goldenseal, saffron, lemons and raw beet juice all activate and clean the liver.

17. Kidneys

Excellent	Good	Fair	Poor
No markings on kidney.	Shadow deeper color than eye	No deterioration or white.	White, infection or brown or black showing deterioration.

For Desired Change: Where infection, same as with acute. Where deterioration, cleansing herbal formula, mild food, uric acid removing herbs such as saffron, dandelion. For healing, juniper herb or juniper oil and cornsilk.

18. Bones – Hypercalcemia osteoporosis:

Excellent	Good	Fair	Poor
No markings showing.	No markings showing.	Inflammation of cornea possible beginning.	Pit-like appearance on body structure (Osteoporosis). gray, glandular appearance either side of pupil.

For Desired Change: Gland involvement, check all glands, related, mild food and cleansing herbs.

19. Eyes:

Excellent	Good	Fair	Poor
No markings	No markings	Shadow inherent showing or white showing infection.	Deterioration showing chronic in color.

For Desired Change: White showing on the eye area would be inflammation. In order to move inflammation all fruit, herb laxatives, enemas and high vitamin C. Where deterioration is showing, mild food diet, cleansing herb formula, vitamin B_1, B_2 and vitamin A. Parsley is one of the richest natural sources of vitamin A, even higher than carrots.

20. Ears:

Excellent	Good	Fair	Poor
No markings	No markings	Shadow inherent showing or white	Deterioration showing chronic in color, showing infection.

For Desired Change: White would be infection or inflammation. Where it is earache, an ice bag to scatter the infection away from ear area. Enemas, fruit diet and laxative herbs which will drag the mucus out of the body. If it is a fungus, mullein herb in a tincture or strong tea or pumpkin seed oil, pumpkin seed or black walnut internally. Often where there is chronic deterioration showing, a parasite line will show also, or a radiation line. Before the mucus so involved can be moved out, the parasites must be killed. Black Walnut and pumpkin seed.

21. Anemia:

Excellent	Good	Fair	Poor
No anemia showing	No anemia showing.	Infection or acute showing too often when not on a cleanse.	Anemia showing anywhere in eye.

For Desired Change: Eye is white most of the time, when not on a cleanse, this indicates too much mucus in the blood, can lead to leukemia. Stop intake of mucus forming foods and treat as a cold. Anemia in small areas of the eye, which looks like the peripheral lines, become obscure; these places indicate too much mucus in the area and a lack of oxygen. If it shows in the brain area, more calcium is necessary to bring oxygen to the brain as well as a good cleanse.

22. Scurf Rim:

Excellent	Good	Fair	Poor
No scurf showing.	No scurf showing. deterioration.	Small, irregular showing no deterioration.	Wide scurf, deterioration

For Desired Change: When the scurf rim shows only a darker color than the color of the eye, this is weakness and will result in an added burden on the internal skin as well as bowel and kidneys. Stimulation of the skin, steam or sweat baths, sun baths, massage or bath brush and a good towel rub. When chronic, mild food, cleansing herbs along with those things listed above.

23. Lymphatic Rosary:

Excellent	Good	Fair	Poor
No markings	No markings.	Few white markings in various places on rosary.	Rosary extending all or much of the circumference of the 6th zone. Chronic in color, even in beginning stages.

For Desired Change: Can develop into Hodgkins disease even if the rosary remains white for too long. Clean entire lymphatic system. Mild food and cleansing herbs, particularly laxatives. Flush the body lymph. When chronic cholesterol, lecithin helps to emulsify and loosen fatty wastes in arteries. Check for lymphatic rosary across bony structures indicating arthritis. Check glands areas, incorrect calcium balance can cause further calcium buildup, hardening arteries.

SUGGESTED WORK CHART
(see next page)

	Excellent	Good	Fair	Poor	Suggested remedy - Remarks
1. Texture					
2. Focus					
3. Heart					
4. Chronic Color - toxicity					
5. Colon & Stomach					
6. Autonomic Wreath					
7. Nerve Rings					
8. Glands					
9. Open Lesions					
10. Closed Lesions					
11. Parasites					
12. Injury					
13. Surgery					
14. Drugs					
15. Acute					
16. Liver - Gallbladder					
17. Kidneys					
18. Bones					
19. Eyes					
20. Ears					
21. Anemia					
22. Scurf rim					
23. Lymphatic Rosary					

Mild Food to Cleanse:

All vegetables and fruits (as much raw as possible)
Fruit juice (canned, raw or frozen)
Soft oil (raw, cold pressed)
All nuts (must be raw)
Honey (raw)
Sprouts (alfalfa, bean, grain)
All starch vegetables must be baked:
squash, potatoes, parsnips, yams

Some Herbs that Detoxify:

Echinacea   Prickley Ash Berries
Gentian   St. John's wort
Catnip   Blue Vervain
Bayberry   Red Clover
Goldenseal Root   Saffron
Irish Moss   Dandelion
Fenugreek   Mandrake
Chickweed   Senna
Comfrey   Cascara Sagrada

Some Herbs to Kill Parasites:

Black Walnut	Cyani Flowers
Pinkroot	Yellowdock
Pumpkin Seeds	Bearfoot root
Pulsatillo	Poke root
Borage	Nettle
Mandrake	Heal all
Tansy	

Semi-fast:

To cleanse in time of famine or limited food supply and still gain adequate nourishment.

> 1 bowl of mush a day, or
> 1 glass of milk, or
> 1 slice of bread (whole wheat).

CHAPTER 3

WHAT'S IN A TESTIMONY

Open minds and listening ears are ever eagerly searching for truth and ways to improve and truly enjoy life. Closed minds and stopped ears are forever locking their doors in the faces of opportunity, progress and peace. Thus do they doom themselves to stagnation, decay and misery.

J. Melvin Gibby
8/13/1961

Like health, happiness, and a good marriage, a testimony is a fleeting thing: you have to work at it to keep it. For brief episodes, as we apply what we have learned, our testimonies of any law – putting our finger in the socket and experiencing a shock, the profound anguish resulting from hateful words – exercises a certain influence on us each living moment. It is, therefore, important that we maintain a good memory bank in our computer brain in order that we may avoid too many mistakes. Even though most mistakes only hurt a little, others can kill us. Too many of us live naïvely inattentive to those things that bring us happiness or pain either in our physical body or in our surroundings. If we were lost in a jungle with wild animals and physical danger, we would become as cunning as a cat, we would give everything we did a little more thought. We would become more aware, logical, and emotional – feeling, thinking, watching, praying, and then acting more correctly for each given situation. Too often when a person has had a beautiful testimony of natural healing methods, the passing of time and a busy schedule lets them slip back into bad habits and they even forget what they did to get better so as to avoid further problems.

> *"Every hardship we encounter in life, if conquered, is a great stepping stone toward our ultimate goal whatever it may be. But unconquered, it remains a persistent stumbling block, which stubbornly impedes our progress until we develop the will and the intelligence to remove it from our path."*
>
> *J. Melvin Gibby*
> *9/6/1961*

A so-called learned man speaking on a talk show recently told how you can tell a quack medical book. He said it would have testimonies. This statement reminds me of Paul before King Agrippa when Festus said, *"Much learning doth make thee mad."* Though Paul was not mad, sometimes much learning seems to make some men of science mad. They forget the testimonies written in the many books of the past have prevented us from reliving the dark ages. All books are testimonies of someone's experience – good or bad; these are the things we learn from. It is our task to search these things out, weigh carefully each witness, and give our whispered prayer to heaven for confirmation, and then proceed accordingly. As you read these testimonies, it will be your prerogative to make a judgment.

> *"Truth is any real and eternal principle that is inalterable by man, time, conditions or even by God himself. Error is a departure in thought, word or deed from the principles of fundamental truth."*
>
> *J. Melvin Gibby*

It should be noted that the following people are from different religious backgrounds and yet the thread of faith in God seems to weave its way through most of their testimonies in their search for truthful answers to their health problems. Far be it for me to take the credit some of these people give to me in these testimonies. All I have done is teach the truth, they picked it up, applied it, and proved it, at least to themselves. For my part I thank the Lord for the knowledge He has given me and the glorious testimony He has given me.

My gratitude also reaches out to all these wonderful people who have had the courage and faith to find these answers.

Ruth Jacobson

Licorice root has been an invaluable aid to me in the treatment of low blood sugar. It has enabled me to carry on throughout the day without the low blood sugar letdown, even if I miss a meal. It has eliminated the fuzzy mind when I just couldn't think, concentrate, or remember. I sleep better, no longer having the "go to bed tired, get up tired" feeling. Now I carry licorice root with me instead of nuts. If I happen to have forgotten to take it, or if I encounter severe stress, a dose of licorice gives me a quick pickup and new energy within a few minutes. I find that diet plays an important part in the effectiveness of licorice root. White sugar and white flour products can wipe out the benefits of the herb. I took time to test this out thoroughly before making my statement. I wanted to be sure I was accurate on it. I just started my son Darrell on it and he was complaining of exhaustion and he is getting the same pickup I do with it.

Myrth Kidd

I would like to add my testimony to those, who like mine have read and put to the test, Mrs. Griffin's book, *Is Any Sick Among You?*. I'm a mother of 10 children, all of them of average good health, at least I have felt this up to our last child. Even though to most people, she seemed to follow a healthy pattern, because she ate well, and was big for her age in stature and weight. This is a mistake many of us make, but my mother's instinct told me all was not well, especially when throat and ear infection became a common thing to her. I knew also, her little body was sluggish, and that her chubbiness was not a good sign of healthiness. I pondered these things in my mind. The doctor told me, and I'm sure he was truthful as far as his knowledge and instruments could tell, that she was fine. So on with the food and antibiotics with some kind of "give her a few years and she'll outgrow it" thought in my mind we went steadily on. About six months before I heard Mrs. Griffin's first lecture, I decided it would be good for me to try some juice fasting and exercise, to sum it all up, try and pull myself together, after all I was 46 with 10 children, and I felt every bit of it. I was amazed how soon I began to see results. It was spring, and as we gardened and gathered asparagus, the truth my mother taught me, for she was a nurse in days when only the herb and natural foods where their medication, "that God, not man produces that which is good for the stomach". That spring and summer prepared me for one of the greatest experiences of my life, the lectures and "the book", as we refer to it at our house, by LaDean Griffin. Not only has it brought a new way of life to me, but my little Heather, whom I spoke of earlier, is like a new child. What a joy it has been to watch her change. No more bottles of antibiotics, because in studying her eyes, I could see her weaknesses. Oh, at first this was frightening, for I could see my fears did have merit, all was not well with her, but then we got with the program, no animal products, no white sugar, no white flour, in fact straight fruits, vegetables, nuts, raw honey and herbs. I watched the change begin to take place both in her eyes and in her whole self, she was almost 3 years old when we started and now some 16 months later I can hardly believe the difference. She still has her inherent weaknesses, but we know this now, and we also know that a healthy, happy life can be hers, if we do not add to her problems. I could tell you many more things about myself but space won't allow, so to those who read my testimony, I bring to you good tidings, it's a great life and because of an old but new knowledge, I am convinced we can enjoy it to its fullest.

LaVerne A. Milam

Herbs working from within the body; chiropractic from without: blood pressure record of Laverne A. Milam age 57, beginning 4/21/75. Record on file in office of a doctor in Alhambra, California.

4-21-1975	160/100	6-3-1975	130/80
5-1-1975	150/90	6-6-1975	130/80
5-8-1975	140/90	6-9-1975	120/80
5-13-1975	135/80	6-13-1975	120/80
5-22-1975	130/80	6-16-1975	120/80
5-28-1975	130/80		
6-20-1975	130/80 (after treatment down to 120/80)		
6-26-1975	140/80 (after treatment down to 130/80)		
7-10-1975	120/80		

Beginning on 4-22-1975, I knew the combination of herbs for high blood pressure was capsicum and garlic, but by mistake I picked the heart combination of Hawthorn berries and capsicum off the shelf in the dim light and without my glasses and started on a plan of two, four times a day; at mealtime and just before bedtime. On my second trip to the doctor, as you can see as of 5-1-1975, it was down. But the doctor was not satisfied. He asked whether I was on the herbs which I had told them I was going to try. I told him, "yes, but it's like this, although I should be having two, four times a day, today for instance, I had two at breakfast, but I wasn't home for lunch, I won't be home for dinner, and in fact, I won't even get home until sometime around 12 tonight." He then informed me I had to do something definite about this, because he wanted it to come down. So I told him, all right I would commence to carry a day's supply in my purse and faithfully use it. Before the next visit to his office, I suddenly discovered I had been taking the wrong combination, but you will notice, since it was for the heart and I had half the correct combination by having capsicum, the pressure had started down. At this point I would like to explain that all my life I have never had a problem with high blood pressure and couldn't believe it when the doctor told me this was high. I really felt tops. I had never had any of the symptoms or warnings most people have; such as flushed face, tingling in hands or legs, tingling in the head or neck. I didn't even know what the normal for me should be. I had never had to be concerned. So the next visit on 5-8-1975, you can see it is still dropping. This was when I asked the doctor what my normal blood pressure should be. So he showed me how you start with the average 20-year-old pressure of 120/80, and for each two years of age after 20, you add one MM is a reading, which made mine for my age to be 138/90. As you can see, my reading for that day was 140/90, about a week and a half after the first reading. Then it occurred to me and I asked the doctor, "Doctor, if all systems in your body are go and you are really feeling great, why should age even enter into the picture? Why shouldn't I be able to reach the level of a 20-year-old?" He just grinned and said, "Listen, you just stay at 138/90 and I'll be happy." As you can see by the above chart, approximately 6 weeks after the first reading, I reached the reading of a 20-year-old and the doctor was amazed.

Mabel U. Ziros

74

I wanted to add my testimony for herbs. The first one I tried was black cohosh one year ago. I have had a complete hysterectomy and one fourth of one breast removed because of fibroid tumors, and have had to take hormone shots. I stayed off hormone shots as long as I could and when I went back for a checkup I was low in hormones and the doctor put me back on them and then after a while he started me on the pill and after a while I started getting the lumps in my breasts, very similar to the problems I had before surgery and I felt very discouraged. I was telling my problem to a friend of mine who was selling herbs and she had your new book, *"Is Any Sick Among You?"*. She said, "Let's check in this book and see which of the herbs is the female hormone." We looked it up and it is black cohosh, and after reading about it I decided to try it, there was nothing to lose, the cost was very little compared to the shots or the pill. I did not know how many capsules to take but this being natural, I was not afraid to take two capsules morning and night, and sometimes at noon. The results have been unbelievable and I do not have the lumps in my breasts, or any of the side effects I had with the shots and the pills. I did not even finish the bottle of pills after I started using the herbs. Mrs. Griffin, before I had a terrible problem with dryness and the doctor said all I could do was use KY jelly, well now I do not have to use that and I am much more comfortable. So I am thankful to my friend and to you for the knowledge I have gained from your books and your lectures on herbs. Now I am using the various herbs for various problems and I have had equally good results. The more I study and learn about herbs, the more thankful I am for the convenience of the herbs we can now get in the capsules.

Elizabeth B. Silver

Having been plagued with psoriasis since high school age and having tried various treatments through the years, I finally, (at age 57) found notable relief in the herb and juice program of Warren Kirley Crosby. I am convinced that following this regime periodically will counteract the flare-up of psoriasis. It may well be that person's able to follow a fresh vegetable and fruit diet etc. as he outlines in a sustained fashion would need the herb-juice treatment less often or not at all. It is a great relief to have come across a successful program of action in treating this disease – without drugs – thanks to Mr. Crosby.

Mr. Crosby

Heart attack July 29, 1974 caused from stress, overwork, strain. Went to the doctor. While he was in the hospital his wife brought him lecithin and vitamin E. Started him on cleansing diet, by October upon recommendation of his general practitioner, went to cardiologist, had full physical, x-rays, blood, urine, treadmill confirmed severe heart attack, gave him Fredrickson diet, walking 2 miles, or 4 miles 10 minutes per mile. Come back in a year. Three months after attack went back to work 40 hours a week, walked 2 miles a day, 2000 units vitamin E, 1000 mg. C, 800 super B, 104 mg. Lecithin, 2 capsules a day nervine herbs, 2 capsules ginseng, 4 saffron.

Recovery: his doctor stated he was probably in better condition now than he has ever been. He said he knows now when he is tired, to go home and rest, not overdue, to be aware of "what I'm doing and what my body is doing". 180 pounds, 6 feet tall, Doctor said lose 6 to 8 pounds, now down to 168.

My dear sister in Christ;

It was a revelation to enjoy your seminar and it ended all too soon. Thanks for the knowledge, and may God bless all your endeavors and keep you healthy and increase your energy. As I promised, the leper photos, for you to use as you see fit and may they impress the doubters, that seem to multiply. It all began 30 years ago last Christmas. I'll be brief, I saw at one time, 80 lepers at the Lepersario Palo Seco, Panama, and it changed my life. Degradation itself and having committed no crime, they are prisoners, behind locked doors and gates for the rest of their lives. When I explained it to my wife, she too got the fever and we searched for 5 1/2 years in Europe and finally discovered the formula on the Island of Rhodes in the Aegean. We were searching for a cure for leprosy only and found among the books, many cures for many things. And recently, Lupus was added to the cures, praise God! Your book may bring hope and release from bondage and I wish you would mention that the same formula will help and in fact, cure Lupus. It is far worse than cancer, as you know and they are helpless and we must help them. Please get in touch with Mrs. Cook, she too, is carrying the torch hopefully, that one day they will all be cured and accept our Lord and Savior. Bless you in your work.

Sincerely,
Kirkley

Irene Hotten

A young girl (28) complaining of menstrual problems and a severe bladder infection. Periods accompanied by severe cramps, flow was black and stringy, bladder infection odorous and passage painful. Reading of eyes showed spots in bladder and ovarian areas. Colon so black and distended it frightened me, huge mass in area of sigmoid flexure. Young lady claimed she was not constipated, that she had regular movements every four or five days!!! She had never had either a colonic or an enema and had to be instructed in the use of the enema bag. A complete change of diet – juices for one week then fresh vegetables and fruits, yogurt and exercise. One month later period started black and changed to red on third day with lessening of cramping. Still cannot get any normal activity of bowel. Second month brought mobility of bowel on its own without enemas. Periods normal red and no cramping. When asked what had happened to the bladder infection she replied, "Oh, I forgot all about it". Eyes showed a cleansing of the entire bowel area but with some residual diverticulas. The relief of the pressure of the huge mass that had been in the sigmoid area releasing the ovary so it could empty following ovulation and allowing the bladder to return to its normal position thereby emptying, entirely cleared up the bladder infection. No drugs, herbs or medicine of any kind were used just common sense!!

Vida Walters

My physical problems began when I was a very young women. As I went from one doctor, to another for help it was diagnosed as anything from nervous stomach to sluggish digestive system. I was always led to believe that the problem was not serious and their diet and medication would help me. Sometimes it did for a few months then all the old symptoms would return. As more and more foods seem to give me distress I was merely asked to delete them from my diet; which was already restricted to mild and bland foods. My condition continued to get worse and there seem to be no place else to go for help. I was tired much of the time and very discouraged; not knowing where I could find someone who could really understand my problem and give me some help. Eventually a method of correct eating habits, using mostly fruits and vegetables, was explained to me. Within a three month period of time I was feeling the effects of this new diet. The stomachaches I had been used to were gone and I had the vitality do things I hadn't enjoyed for years. This was over 3 1/2 years ago and I am still happy with the program and am grateful for those responsible for helping me. My entire family has benefited from my experience and have learned to see the value of good eating habits and we are grateful for the good health that we are enjoying.

Life was spared

My life was spared for the second time in two years. On Thursday, October 30, I had a dry tickly throat. I started right away sucking vitamin C and went to a meeting in Taylorsville, down by Salt Lake City to hear Stan Malstrom speak. I had a car load that wanted to go down, I had a 20-year-old girl from rock Springs with multiple sclerosis, who wanted to go so bad. She was going to school in Salt Lake City, I was to pick her up there and take her to the meeting, which I had taped and is very beautiful. The next day I was sick and stayed in bed all day Friday, and until noon Saturday, felt better, got up at that time to go to a meeting I had scheduled in Hillyard I felt was another must. I came right home and went to bed and stayed there till 2:00 Sunday. I had a kitchen to draw for my husband which I went to the home of the Browns and did this, by 5:30 I was really sick again so I told Raymond, my husband, I felt I needed to go to the hospital. Upon arriving there, I was asked how long I had been sick, I said this was the third day. The nurse told me not to expect the doctor to come to me then, they only came on the first day of an illness. I tried to explain I thought I had strep throat, I couldn't breathe and my right gland was as large as when you had mumps. The nurse looked in my throat, called the doctor, said it was a little red.

My husband talked with the doctor, he said go home and take a couple of aspirin, gargle then swallow it. I was horrified, I knew aspirin would have choked me to death. The nurse said before this to take vinegar and salt and water and gargle which I did that night I sat up all night. Every time I tried to lay my head down I felt I was strangled to death. I also had been taking goldenseal and comfrey and fenugreek, but by 3:00 I knew that unless that mucus started to drain I was doomed. I read in *Natures Medicine Chest* No. 2, a part on sore throat with cayenne pepper in a tea. I at once started to take the tea and right away the mucus started to break up, only in little pieces.

By the next morning I was very, very sick. My husband had to go to Salt Lake, so as soon as my son got home from school at noon, I had him drive me to the clinic and the doctor took me right in and said I should go right into the hospital or I can be treated at home with saltwater gargle every hour. He gave me a shot of penicillin, I went home and did what he said and was a very sick person. I was spitting up every few seconds but still I could not lay down and breathe. That day my girlfriend called and said to take slippery elm in a tea which I did, this helped the mucus flow some. By the time my husband was home at 5:00 I was still unable to breathe only sitting up. He asked if I wanted to be taken to the hospital. I said I felt that I would like the priesthood to bless me. He went right to the phone and called our home teacher, he picked up our bishop and gave me a beautiful blessing. At this time my girlfriend brought me some penny royal, she put some in water in an electric fry pan set it in the bathtub and I was instructed to open my mouth and breathe it. It relaxed my throat so at 3:00 in the morning I was able to lay down but I couldn't sleep a bit on the couch or anywhere, I finally lay down by my husband and was able to relax and sleep for one hour. By the next day I felt well on the way to recovery. I remember as a child when I had my throat like this I was ill for at least two or three weeks, this time I was really ill, badly, for only three days, isn't that a beautiful testimony? When you take vitamins and herbs, your body is on more of a condition to throw off disease than when it is run down and not able to heal itself.

Problem solved with mild foods

I have for a long time had real hate feelings towards my husband when he didn't do exactly as I wanted him to. I also had no desire for any intimate contact. These things have completely gone when I remain on mild foods with iodine, licorice and chlorophyll. I would, whenever under stress at all, wake up each morning as if I had a bad head cold coming on. My nose was stuffy and would burn to the point of being quite painful. I would also have burning eyes and the feeling of a partial earache. When I stay on the mild foods I don't have this problem any longer. Before I started on the mild food program I had continual backache. After I was on the mild food and no herbs but licorice for about two weeks, my backache left and only when I go back to eating concentrated foods do I get the backache again.

Previous to going on the mild foods, my feet were so rough that I couldn't put on my nylon stockings. The skin would snag when I went barefoot and rip and bleed. Since being on the mild foods (it took about eight weeks), my feet became as smooth as silk and have remained this way. Many times I have given my children lobelia with cayenne, when sick to the stomach. Whether they vomit or not doesn't seem to matter but in a couple of hours after sleep, they feel completely well.

Doyle Walters

I have a testimony of the healing power of herbs, mild foods and vitamins. I had a duodenal ulcer build scar tissue and stop the flow of food out of the stomach. The stoppage was critical and would have required surgery resulting in the removal of two thirds of the stomach, but with the use of herbs, vegetable juices and vitamin E, I was able to bring this condition under control.

This was not an easy thing for me to do. It required tremendous willpower but the results were well worth the effort. I am 40 pounds lighter, my energy is way up and a sick day is almost nonexistent.

Ruth Ruhland – Diary on a healing crisis – picture see page 45

Skinny formula – started May 7 on "000" size, three per day and I went to 12 one day, but mostly 6 to 9. May 9 my neck and head hurt me so bad I went for an adjustment. I had cramping and went to the bathroom often, about 6 to 10 times. One black stool on the evening of May 10. May 13 had another adjustment, my right side of neck and my right ear were so sore I could hardly touch, my ear started a yellow discharge, rather hard, now July 12 it is about clear. My desire for food has lessened and I'm not hungry. May 14 my neck on the right side is so bad I can't move it. My heart picked up a few extra beats in the morning. Last night (May 13) I went sound asleep and really relaxed. I had three hours of sound sleep, woke at 6:30 but wanted to lay in bed. I just couldn't get going until noon. June 3, I've got a lump on my head right above my spine. It's so sore, I can't lay on my back in bed and can hardly move my neck. The glands are swollen on both sides of it, about one inch away. The desire for food has really gone. I could eat once a day to keep from being so dizzy. June 10, the lump is gone and now I'm having eye trouble, can't see to read even with glasses. My far vision is okay, it's only close. My heart picked up a couple of beats but seems okay. Under both my arms and right legs I have large lumps and pus and blood. This lasted 10 days and went away but came open and drained. My bowels are still loose (June 20) and I'm on nine a day. I'm 6 pounds lighter, and was away for dinner the other night and got ill when I was served a steak. I had to go vomit. I crave juice, so I'm making carrot juice I can't stand coffee (that's unusual).

July 9, so sick, so awful sick, have had a headache across the back for last three days, the most awful sore throat, and aching, strange feelings down my legs as I lay in bed. My eyes have gotten better. I passed strings of blood, and fresh blood in the urine.

July 10, pus came out in the urine on its own. I had a very difficult time urinating until the pus and dark strings came out of the bladder. Others were clear as I put a tampon in to be sure. I really worked to get strings and plus. I believe a tea cup of pus. I believe my bladder is tipped again. I felt like I was going to die. My right side of nose drained pus, and I've lost my voice. The left side started today, July 12, to be clogged. I had 103 temperature and July 11, at night I soaked my pajamas three times and had to change. The bathwater was oily or real different this morning. My urine is clear but I'm hoarse and feel like I have congestion in my lungs. I'm drinking grape juice, I'm really bloated, my eyelids are so swollen and I feel terrible. Tomorrow I'll stay in bed. I'm on goldenseal, half teaspoon three times a day with 1 teaspoon of licorice each time. I just ate a pint of strawberries today, I was so hungry for them. Weight loss 8 pounds, even bloated. I feel terrible tonight but this is best I can report.

I'm still on the herbs. My nose is all hard and yellow inside but I use cream on it. I really had no sharp pains, my headache is dull now and the most distress was on right side where the gallbladder came out, I did hurt terrible in there. I found it very difficult to breathe, yesterday especially. I do believe I had a crisis. I had a total jet black stool on the ninth, the fluid with this tool was even black. I feel better and I'm sure Sunday in bed all day will help.

* * *

Ruth told me how much better she felt after this cleansing crisis and she looked better than I have seen her in several years. As you can observe, the healing crisis only lasted two or three days we can have the good and bad days up until the crisis, while the waste is eliminating on the bad days, a little at a time until we eventually reach the point where the body vitality is sufficient to experience a healing crisis.

Problem solved with mild food

At the time I was studying and taking classes from LaDean, I conversed with my sister about what I was learning. Because of my studies in iridology I began to notice people's eyes and my sister's eyes were particularly interesting to me because she had one or two dark spots in the iris. I hesitated to talk to her about them, not knowing how she would accept it. After a few weeks I observed that one spot became larger and very dark. My sister had complained of back problems and pain which she suspected to be gallbladder. Her doctor, after x-rays and checkup, told her he could offer no help or determination as to what the problem was or what to do with it so to let it go for a time. The spot grew larger, it was located in the right iris beginning in the ascending colon area and spread up into the shoulder area. The pain was in the upper right side of her back under the shoulder.

After hearing in class about a man with a similar problem and what he had done for it, I suggested to my sister to go on a mild food diet, take psyllium seed powder in water with laxative every night and also take a high enema each day for at least three days. She continued with this treatment for two weeks she noted the spot in her eye had faded she told me she thought she had passed a bowel impaction. When I saw her after two weeks I detected no spot left in that area of her eye (iris).

Hearing helped

1. Chiropractic adjustments
2. Special blessing
3. Apple juice three-day cleanse
4. Full mild foods, three months
5. Herbs, cayenne, apple cider vinegar, the vitamins, started passing chunks of old mucus.

Cleared throat and spit out a large chunk apparently from the Eustachian canal judging from its shape, after that, level of hearing went up, old aid defective, used alone or only need on low level to hear. Other benefits; chronic, rotten breath gone, asthma mucus condition gone, hair starting to grow in, teeth start to bother, trip to dentist revealed four impacted teeth, after removal hearing on right side went up noticeably. Age 40, deaf since six months of age. 1963 complete ear test, hearing loss so pronounced, both ears, hearing aid useless. Nerves conducting messages to brain dead. 1965, suffered back injury, series of chiropractic adjustments, following this, hearing came in for a few seconds at a time over a period of weeks, very spastic. 1970, hearing test again, hearing level in left year in the low range, other ear no response. 1972 – 73 went on mild foods, discontinued as too expensive, went on vegetable diet, took LaDean's advanced iridology class, began in earnest, went on full program.

Children helped with herbs

My 11 month old baby had had a bad cold for over two weeks, but with juices, garlic enemas, and lots of vitamin C, we had been able to stay just ahead of it. One night, in the middle of the night, I was awakened with the kind of creepy cough that makes one jump straight out of bed. I went in to him and his breathing was really labored. I took him in the kitchen to look at him, to keep from waking my daughter. He was obviously running a high fever. I was shocked at the way his face was swollen. His eyes and cheeks were puffy, I thought, "Oh no, we better get him to the hospital fast." As I left the kitchen to go into my bedroom to wake my husband, the word "Lobelia" came to me. I ignored it, and again I felt, "Lobelia". A week earlier, I had asked a good friend what I could do to help my baby, in addition to suggesting garlic enemas, she had brought me a few Lobelia capsules. When she gave them to me, I thought "No way". I had read in several books the drastic results that came from using Lobelia. When the feeling came to me the third time, I turned and went back into the kitchen. I thought, "It's now or never". I took half the capsule and mixed it with a little honey and put it in my baby's mouth. Neither of us was prepared for what happened. Within a few seconds, he threw up a big mouthful of mucus and phlegm. There was a large beach towel on the back of one of the dining room chairs, my children had been playing with earlier, and I grabbed it to have the baby spit up in. I no more than folded it over, then he did it again. Each time, he would catch his breath, then up would come some more. He began sneezing, his eyes were running and he broke out in heavy perspiration all over. He continued this way for about 15 minutes. When he got through, he was wet all over. I was shaking like a leaf, but had had a deep calming feeling that I was doing what was right, and that everything would be okay. When he finally quit, I looked at his eyes, to see if he was okay. He smiled at me, and in a few minutes was down running all over the house. After I recovered, I made him some peppermint leaf tea, and rocked him to sleep to make sure he was okay. He didn't cough again that night, and within a few days was completely well.

Another time, my 11-year-old daughter came from school complaining of a bad upset stomach. Her face was flushed and feverish and it was obvious she didn't feel well. I headed for the enema bag, and she said, "Not that, give me a lobelia, instead". So I did. Within a few minutes, she threw up, went to bed that night feeling better and got up and went to school the next day. I'm convinced we got the infection while it was still in her stomach and before it had spread to her intestines and on through her body. Needless to say, lobelia has become a much used herb in our home. We agree completely, that it is the "intelligence" herb. It goes where it is needed and does the job that must be done. It's results are very different each time, depending on what the person using it needs.

Denice Stokes

It is not just a figure of speech, when I say, "I'll be eternally grateful." After my second baby was born, my health, daily deteriorated. I had pain in my abdomen, and the pain in my back became worse with each passing day. Doctors said x-rays show nothing in abdomen, and finally concluded it was arthritis in my back. Also, I was diagnosed to have geographic tongue. To make things worse, my new baby seemed horribly unhappy. I stayed awake nights listening to his raspy breathing, and checking to see if he had rolled over, because when he laid on an arm or hand it would soon turn black. Doctor said; "Oh he'll grow out of it." My nerves were raw, and I was at a loss. No one was able to help. Doctors acted as if they didn't care. I asked myself many times why I had to resign myself to bad health. My patriarchal blessing said, I had a strong, healthy body filled with vigor and vitality. Something went wrong! I asked my heavenly father to help me. My burdensome, unhealthy body was making me a crummy wife, mother, friend, and child of God. The Lord began to open doors. And the best thing of all, LaDean's book; *Is Any Sick Among You?*. It seemed to make sense. And as I began her diet, and felt my Heavenly Father's presence. My heart and spirit were alive with enthusiasm, (a feeling I hadn't had for a long time). Within three days after beginning the diet, my arthritis pain disappeared. I noticed my tongue became normal if I didn't eat meat and salt. I woke at 3 o'clock in the morning, after I had been on the diet about two months. I was in horrible pain in the abdomen area. I could hardly move. Seven o'clock the pain subsided. I passed a very large group of worms all tangled together and then mucus. My baby (nursing from my improved milk) began to act better within two weeks. Every day he passes old filth and mucus, and sometimes parasites. When he gets an earache or a cold, I doctor him with herbs. We are not only saving money, but those unnerving hours spent in the doctor's office. My big treat is to examine my eyes at the end of each day. There are filled with healing white and are surely turning a heavenly blue color. I feel I've been rewarded tenfold for sticking to the diet. October 5, had another crisis, October 16, I passed horrible looking stuff. Baby also had crisis (I think), I can feel my arthritis pain moving out!

Paul and Vee Hull

Following is a short synopsis of some of our healing experiences: I have suffered from eczema over all of my body since I was in third grade after having been given sulfur baths and sulfur salve. I was approximately 41 years old when we changed our diet and stopped all chemical medications. After about one year of no chemicals, I took medication for a kidney infection, my eczema broke out in fury. On another occasion I took aspirin and received the same reaction. We decided at this time to find the right herb for anything we needed for healing. I am entirely free from eczema now. I received a third degree burn on my hand and by immediately using aloe vera gel and vitamin E, I completely healed my hand in two weeks with no scarring. New skin formed under the dead white skin and the damage skin just thinned out and disappeared. At a later date I fell on the back of a metal chair and broke two ribs. By using comfrey and a poultice which I have learned to make, my ribs healed totally in two weeks with no scar ridge in the bone and no further pain. I didn't miss even one day's work and some of my associates said they wouldn't believe they were broken if I hadn't had them x-rayed.

Our daughter had her wisdom teeth pulled and instead of using the antibiotics and pain killers we used vitamin B complex and calcium for the pain, vitamin C to pull out infection and a solution of goldenseal and myrrh as hot as she could take which she held in her mouth to heal the incision and prevent the swelling. She woke up the next morning with no swelling no bleeding and no pain.

Paul had critical health most of his life. His eye showed severe inherent lesions and a starburst colon. He couldn't exercise as it fatigued him and made his muscles ache. He discovered through iridology that he had Addison's disease and with the information in LaDean's book we have seen improvement in his health over the past two years. Just recently his health has taken a dramatic turn for the better and for the first time in his life he can work long hours without fatigue and without muscle soreness. We have a testimony that what LaDean is teaching is the Word of Wisdom as the Lord would have us live and through following the basic principles we have received those "Hidden treasures of knowledge" regarding our own family's health that are promised in the Word of Wisdom. My husband Paul and I have both had serious health problems when we met, married and combined six children from previous marriages, we also had health problems with her children. We were both interested in health through herbs, nutrition and eliminating preservatives in our diet, so we went at it wholeheartedly. We first took salt out of our diet – gradually so the children did not know the difference. It was not until they visited their grandmother and wondered what was wrong with the cereal that we told them that they had not been eating salt. We next switched from sugar to honey and from white bread to sprouted wheat. As we eliminated the preservatives, used more fruits and vegetables, stopped frying, reduced our meat intake and learned to use herbs instead of chemical medications, we found exciting health changes. Our oldest daughter had chronic infections which kept her in and out of school about six weeks a year. She was given high doses of antibiotics to "burn" the infection out of her system and gamma globulin shots to help with the infection. The hours of hospital testing gave no answer as to the cause or any solution to ending the treatment. After Paul and I were married and changed her diet, her health straightened out, she ended her sleepless nights, kept good attendance at school and lost the white pallor to her skin. Her hair, which she was told would have to stay short, grew long and beautiful and her stooped posture straightened up. Our younger son plagued since infancy with constant tonsillitis, regained his health on our new diet and hasn't had a reoccurrence in five years.

At the time we started our diet change, we searched for information on herbs but found it very limited in our area in 1970. We were told of LaDean Griffin's class about 2 1/2 years ago. We both attended and received information that changed our lives and our health. I have a testimony that we were led to LaDean and that she teaches by the spirit. In LaDean's class we learned of the mild food diet and I immediately started using it. Within two weeks I had a healing crisis in the colon I had a forceful cleanse which lasted all night but by morning I felt as though atmospheric pressure had been taken from me. There was no effort in doing anything. Paul and I observed the mild food diet faithfully for over three months. At the end of July we went to a family reunion and my 25th class reunion – both the same day, and ate what was served. I ended up flat on my back, sicker than I remember being for years with a cold, the first sinus infection I have ever had and lung congestion. I learned that my system could no longer tolerate the preservatives in food or the bad combination. Paul and I signed up for LaDean's advanced iridology class and at this time Paul developed a method of photographing the eye for LaDean's classes since that time we have continued to do eye photography, learn iridology and increase our knowledge of herbs and healing

Karen Biddulph

I can't remember a time in my life when I wasn't plagued by bad health. Even as a youth I didn't seem to have the health and vitality that my friends had. In my high school years I had the same problems. After I was married and began to have my family, my health steadily deteriorated until about five years ago, I was plagued constantly with heavy depressions and illness. The depressions were so bad that I constantly feared death and I feared any disease. Any ache or pain was played up in my mind to be a terminal illness, and I would constantly live in fear of death. I had times of depression that I just didn't seem to be able to overcome. Along with this I had a physical problem and I checked with the doctor many times and was only given tranquilizers to keep myself from worrying about it. It got so bad that I couldn't drink water without my stomach hurting. I couldn't eat any food. I had constant pain in my spine and I had headaches that would never stop and of course, the depression came right along. After the birth of my fifth child, I didn't have the energy to even take care of my family. I'd watch all day as the children would run around in their pajamas. I wasn't able to take care my home, and I wasn't able to take care my church responsibilities. Sometimes I'd wonder if my husband and my family might not be better off if I were dead. I was told at this time by my doctor that the best thing I could do for my depression was to see a psychiatrist, and I was almost ready to but I sought help from some church leaders and I was told that psychiatry wasn't the answer to my problem, and that if I'd be faithful, my Heavenly Father would come to my aid and help me out of this problem I was so deeply involved in. So, I begin fasting with my husband and praying that my Heavenly Father might see fit to bless me. I've a firm conviction that all laws which we gain in this life are predicated upon obedience to the principles on which this law is based, and I prayed with all my heart and my soul that my Heavenly Father may see fit to give me this law. In the meantime, I studied the program theory. I studied all the books I could read on nutrition and health. I tried the vitamin supplements. I tried the strong protein drinks and the high protein diet until at last I felt my head was just like a big pumpkin askew on my shoulder. I couldn't even hold my head up at times. My scalp hurt so badly that it even hurt to lie in bed and of course, the depression became worse and worse, till I felt that I was at the bottom of a black pit and couldn't even see the top. After about a year of constantly praying and asking my Heavenly Father to help me, during this time I asked if I should go to a clinic or follow the Orthodox medical route and always I felt inspired that I should not do this. I have a very strong admiration for the medical profession and some of the things which they accomplish and I am grateful they are here for things which we can depend on them for, but in my own particular situation I felt this was not the answer. After a year of this searching, I was told about a series of lectures that were being given not far from our home by LaDean Griffin. A friend of mine said that she would pick me up and take me down to hear the lectures if I would go. Before I went, I stepped into my bedroom and knelt and asked if the Lord could please in some way help me that I wouldn't fear disease. The fear of disease seem to be the cause of a lot of my depression. As I sat listening to Mrs. Griffin lecture, the tears rolled down my cheeks because one of the first things she said was, after we learned things, she would teach us we would no longer have to fear disease, and I felt this was a direct answer to my prayer. I listened to the lectures completely and I had a firm conviction that they were true. When we studied the part on iridology, I was afraid because after looking in my eyes I can see that there were many parts of my body that were deeply diseased and that it would take a lot of dedication and faith to live the program as I should in order to get well. I came home and explained everything that I'd learn to my husband, and he immediately knew that it was true, so our entire family went on the program. We changed our diet to that of mild food. We began taking the herbs that we needed, and we began to take the vitamin supplements, and all those things that we had been taught, to the best of our ability. The results were almost remarkable. We had a little boy who was 18 months old, who had been on Gamma globulin since he was six months old. When he was four days old, we took him into the doctor with a terrible sore throat inflammation and from then until he was eight months old it was a constant round of Gamma globulin, antibiotics, and hospitalization for different diseases. After just three weeks on the mild food diet, he was able to stop all of his Gamma globulin shots which we had been giving to him every six days. He hasn't had a shot now for two years. He's a healthy little boy and he's growing stronger and stronger. Knowing what I do about iridology, looking into his eyes, it's a miracle that we found this program for him, as well as for myself.

During the first year of living on the program, I had a baby – a beautiful little boy, and he's the picture of health, he's strong. His resistance to disease seems to be almost unbelievable. He's an intelligent little baby, and we're very grateful to have him. The rest of our family, also, is showing great improvement in their health. I must admit that during those two years I've had many bad days, and only knowing that this program is true and the testimony which my Heavenly Father has seen fit to give me, has sustained me through some of the bad days. I went several weeks many times without having a good day. I'm finding now after two years that the good days are outweighing the bad days and I have a strength and vitality which I didn't think I would ever have. Another thing that I'm grateful for is that I've been able to get well here with my family. As I've recovered from the illness which was in my body, I've been able to take care of my family and do the things which I could. Another thing which I'd like to mention that Mrs. Griffin taught to us, which is as important as anything that she taught us, was that it's possible to be able to listen to the Spirit and have the Spirit guide and direct us in all the things we do. We've had many experiences, my husband and I, of having a sick child and after administering to him, knowing instinctively what to do and being guided by the Spirit what to do for our children and having them respond almost miraculously to the things which we were told to do. We've taken our children through colds and fevers, ear infection and many different, minor illnesses, and we've been able to take care of them without having to take any antibiotics, and we've known which herbs and which vitamins and what kind of therapy we should give them. The blessing that has been most important to us is knowing that our Heavenly Father lives and that He's willing to give us His Spirit to guide us in the things which we should do for our family. We've learned iridology. We've been privileged to take the advanced classes in iridology, and it is remarkable and further testimony to us that this is true because everything, as we looked into our eyes, corresponded to places that we had been having trouble in our bodies and after two years on the program, it's a miracle to see how our problem areas in her eyes are interlaced with the healing lines which Mrs. Griffin promised would come if we were faithful to the program. It is our testimony as a family these things are true. They have brought nothing but goodness to us. They have brought nothing but peace and harmony in our home and feelings which we have not had in our home until this time. There have been many among our associates who have looked down upon us and ridiculed us and called us fanatics for the things which we have done but we feel that we been following the course which are Heavenly Father would have us take in healing our bodies and becoming more spiritually in tune with Him and living the way that He would have us live. The colds, flu and the illnesses which our family suffered have been the result of living on the program. They are healing crises rather than actual disease crises. Our family has been strict, and I've seen rewards come from living on the program the way that we've done.

Kent Biddulph

My wife Karen has already explained the circumstances in which we became acquainted with the mild food and herbal remedies program as taught by LaDean Griffin. This program has been an answer to our prayers for improved health. Even though it may not be the ultimate in what our Heavenly Father intends, it is a considerable and sizable step above the conventional diet of the general American populace which is accepted by the medical profession to be correct. This viewpoint I cannot accept. I have not taken all of LaDean's classes as my wife has, but I do know this program is correct and follows all scriptural references I have been able to find and study on the subject. In my own way I have tested this program on myself and found very definitely that if I follow the program as outlined, my health, mental attitude and spiritual growth is greatly increased. If I do not follow the program, I do not enjoy the benefits. My experiences after two years of living and eating as taught in the mild foods program and seeking our Heavenly Fathers guidance, reaffirms to me that this program has indeed been an answer to our prayers for our family. I can give my personal testimony of its worth and the truthfulness of the program. I know it can help anyone who seeks after truth and good health.

Marilyn Parkinson (Mr. and Mrs. Bob Parkinson)

We are thankful for the opportunity to leave our witness, along with many others, in this book. We have watched our eyes change through following the mild food diet and through use of herbs. We would encourage anyone who has a desire to be self-sustaining and independent to study iridology and make use of it in caring for their families. In this day of rising medical costs, strikes and shortages, it is encouraging to know that there are simple and practical and inexpensive answers to many of our problems. Thanks to LaDean Griffin for the effort that she has put forth to bring these truths to us.

For Tanyet McKenzie

She was seven months old at the time the program was starting. I was nursing her at this time when I went on the mild foods, and soon after this she began a real cleanse. She had been an extremely nervous baby. She wouldn't sleep at night, she cried continually, someone had to tend her all the time, and yet she seemed to be healthy. During this time I managed to get some of the nervine herbs down her and tried to take all the things away from her that would cause this nervousness. This, in itself, didn't seem to make much difference. But as I increased my licorice root intake, this helped some and then I put her on alfalfa in the form of liquid chlorophyll. At the time I did this, within two days she was like another baby. She quit crying all the time, would sit down and play, and before that she had been so tense and so nervous that when we tried to give her an enema or anything of this kind she would cry and be so upset that we simply couldn't do this, she would just close off. There was no way to get water into her. But after this and she calmed down, then we would give her enemas and we started moving things from her, and we can tell by looking at her eyes, even though we hadn't had a good picture before, that they began to change. I thought that they were almost a black-blue color, but as this began to move the toxic waste, she started to feel better, her eyes are gradually getting to be a lighter blue and she continues to pass an awful lot of waste, far more than the amount of food she eats. At this time she is sleeping through the night, she is happy for the most part and she has color back in her face, her eyes don't have the dark look that was around them, and I contribute it more than anything to the mild foods and liquid chlorophyll.

Cheri Munns

My daughter May was four months old and I was having a hard time nursing her, as with my first baby. Up until six weeks after I gave birth, nursing worked beautifully but then I would start my period and nursing became a problem. I hadn't started May on any solids or bottles, so that wasn't causing my problem. I did everything my breast-feeding book said but with no results. Well, I was becoming a nervous wreck and my daughter started sucking her thumb to fall to sleep since my nursing her every half hour around-the-clock didn't satisfy her. I was convinced giving her cereal wasn't the answer, so I poured my heart out to my Heavenly Father to know what the answer was. Why were many young mothers nursing their babies so easily while others like myself were having such a struggle? I got so desperate that I threatened the Lord that if I wasn't able to nurse my daughter the way I knew nature had intended I wouldn't have any more children. This was quite a threat for me because I had always wanted a dozen children or more if I possibly could. Well, my prayers were answered when the manager of the apartment complex we lived in brought iridology into our conversation one day and then told me about the mild food diet and the reasons behind it. I then read the book, *Is Any Sick Among You?*, And after living on the mild food diet for two weeks, I was able to satisfy my baby with more milk and an easier letdown. After another month on the diet I stopped having periods; the way nature intended to have birth control. My girl is now one and a half years old and I'm still nursing her beautifully. I thank my Father in Heaven every day for the wonderful blessing of health this new way of eating is brought to my entire family with the added help of herbs.

Healing crisis

After being on the mild food diet for about six months and thinking I would never have a big healing crisis, it happened! At first I thought that I had caught the flu. I ran to the bathroom all morning and then it really hit, like being in labor. I had severe abdominal cramps, except they wouldn't let up. My diarrhea turned pink which I assumed was watered down blood with mucus in it. After a while no more blood, only straight white mucus which turned yellow, green brown and then to my utter horror, greenish black which came out in globs. Before this crisis I had trouble with foul-smelling gas whenever I ate dried figs, dates, raisins or avocados. After my crisis, they never bothered me again to eat them. I feel that the crisis I experienced cleaned my whole bowel out of all that morbid mucus waste that had probably been there most of my life! It was well worth the pain to be that much further on the road to perfect health.

Mariphyllis Foreman

I had melanoma cancer and the doctor wanted me to have surgery. I decided first to try herbs. I took comfrey and blue violet leaves, put them in the blender with honey and lemon, I drank 10 to 12 glasses a day for two weeks, and then went 3 to 4 months on raw food. After that length of time I went to the Cancer Clinic in Mexico and they found no trace of cancer

Rhona S. Hanks

I'm a member of the Church of Jesus Christ of Latter-day Saints. About 3 1/2 years ago, I became very interested in studying the 89th section of the Doctrine and Covenants where the Lord gives His people some guidelines for good health. I came to the conclusion that there were many things contained in this section that were far above my level of understanding.

A well-meaning Sunday School teacher of mine when I was a child, told our class that herbs were vegetables. I didn't question that statement until I was 30 years old. I made it a matter of fasting and praying to my Father in Heaven for answers to my questions about good health and to increase my knowledge of the Word of Wisdom. Within a few weeks, I was inspired to study other books concerning the uses of herbs in healing the body and more correct foods to feed my family. From this information, my husband and I decided to try some of the things.

Our youngest boy who is eight years old, has been sickly since birth with one thing or another. For the past two years, we have tried to feed him as many fresh fruits and vegetables as possible, as well as fresh raw vegetable juices. We have cut down on his intake of sugar, refined flour, and meat. We have added vitamins, minerals, and herbs to his daily diet. Last year in the second grade, he only missed 2 1/2 days of school because of illness. We have been so thrilled; that is a fantastic achievement for him.

From LaDean Griffin's lectures on health, I learned about the purge for the gallbladder. My husband had been having what our doctor suspected was trouble with his gallbladder for several years. I had had my diseased gallbladder removed at the age of 22, and my husband knew well the difficulty and expense of that kind of operation. He decided to try the purge. He passed so many stones the next day that we stopped trying to count them, they were in varying sizes and in many shades of green. We estimated that there were over 2 cupfuls of stones. Since that time, which has been three years, he has not experienced any more related symptoms.

For over three years, I've been telling myself that the mild food diet was for sick people. If I ever got really sick, I'd try it. I finally quit rationalizing, stirred up my courage, and went on the mild food diet three weeks ago. Granted this is too short of a time to test it, but this much I can say, not only do I feel good, I am losing weight in the process, I'm beginning to feel a part of the sensation that comes with self-mastery.

Whether it is putting goldenseal on a cut finger or treating the flu with mild food and herbs, our family has been truly blessed with this knowledge. It is my testimony that the Lord answered my prayers and directed me to these truths.

Tumor passed on mild food

We are blessed to have many children, but it was disappointing to my husband and I when I lost a baby about two months along. I then heard about and read LaDean's book and started on a mild food diet. A few months later I was pregnant again. I began taking herbs when a bleeding problem developed. Just past two months I lost this baby at home. I felt so bad, but still I had a peaceful feeling. A few minutes later I was impressed to know that I wasn't through I began to bear down and passed a long tumor.. What a blessing to see health returning to my body.

Teresa Clinger

Thank you for the love and understanding that you have for everyone. You're so beautiful, and I love you so very much. I hope with all my heart that I can learn to be as loving and beautifully spiritual as you are. I knew from the first time that I met you that my prayers had been answered. I'm so thankful that I am a daughter of my Father in Heaven and for some of the understandings I have of Him. I plan to learn a great deal more so that I may be able to raise my children to walk uprightly before our Father in Heaven. The only thing that is strongly planted in my mind is to teach them to know while they are just little to take, and live with the herbs and mild food so that soon, some day, they may be able to walk uprightly before our Father in Heaven. It's hard to imagine how wonderful it would be and I want my children to be part of this. I came to know of the herbs and mild foods when my baby was born. He was born October 22, 1974. When they put this baby in my arms, I knew there was something wrong. He was perfect physically but I didn't really pay too much attention to the warnings I had then because I didn't know too much about the mild food and herbs, but after two weeks had gone by, I knew I had to do something. I took him to my doctor, and I told him I needed some help. There was something wrong. I told the doctor he acted as though he was in great pain.

He slept beautifully for a week and from that day on it seemed as if he was going downhill. He couldn't sleep. He had a hard time breathing. He was so white and so limp. I have a little girl three years old, and I know how a newborn is supposed to respond and grow. The doctor sent me home with two big pockets of prescriptions and changed the baby's milk to a formula – soybean milk. I gave him his prescription and milk for a month. There was no change. Now he could hardly lift his head at all. It seemed when I prayed to my Father in Heaven I couldn't pray without soaking the sheets with tears. I prayed so hard that He would answer my prayers.

After that, I took my baby to the Idaho Falls doctor. He put him in the Idaho Falls Hospital for a week. They x-rayed every organ in his body and took lab tests. There was still no change. The doctor still didn't know what was wrong, he put him in my arms, and he said," I guess it's just because he's so used to the attention he gets," so he told me to take him home and put him in a room and let him cry.

I took him home and I gave him a mother's blessing and when Dee got home that night, we got everyone together and gave him another blessing and that night he had no trouble sleeping, and I was able to sleep myself

The next day my mother had talked to a lady about mild foods and herbs and my prayers have been answered I was ready to do anything because I knew my baby was dying. We had his eyes read, (they were a natural blue), they were such a dark brown that the parasites sunburst and the deterioration had turned them so dark you could hardly see the pupil. We put them on fruits and mild herbs and through fasting and prayer I have a live and happy baby. After five weeks of herbs and fruits, he started expelling tumors, things that you would never dream would come out of a pure, perfect, newborn baby. I knew my Father in Heaven was close and my babies little body just beamed. I knew I was doing the right thing.

When I held this baby I felt so close to my Father in Heaven. I haven't been to a doctor since December. He still has a long way to go, but he is alive and well. His eyes are starting to turn a light blue. I have never in all my life seen anything so wonderful, so spiritual as the herbs and mild foods. It has brought our family so close to our Father in Heaven.

Verlyn Ritchason

I have had a thyroid (goiter) problem for nine years. I've tried half grain of thyroid medicine, about 8 1/2 years ago. I used it for about one week and it made me very nervous, so I quit using it. About three years later a health food store owner told me about kelp so I took about six small kelp tablets for a week – then I was very nervous so I quit taking that. Then the thyroid enlarged and started hurting. Then I took an herb combination of Irish Moss, kelp, parsley and capsicum – I took one the first day – it made my thyroid hurt – none the second day – one the third day – a little hurting – none the fourth day – one the fifth day – no hurting. I have been taking one or two every day since March. The goiter has diminished to half the size and no hurting. I feel great!

Georgia Stephenson

My name is Georgia Stephenson. I live in Orem, Utah. Last August 1974, I attended a class given by Mrs. Griffin on her book, *Is Any Sick Among You?*. I have recently, over the last three years, been interested in health and felt there were many things about health that the average person didn't know.

I went to her class after reading her book and was somewhat skeptical about some of her ideas concerning health and illness. I had never been what you really could consider is sick or sickly person. I've never had anything really seriously wrong with me, but I have had very troublesome acne since about 12 years old. I have spent a lot of money on dermatologists, etc., with not much help from them. I have also been a good 30 pounds overweight for about seven years and have tried every diet that has ever been thought up.

After attending Mrs. Griffin's class I decided to try mild food and some herbs. I have always been a nervous person and unable to stand much stress. I started right on mild food without any problem at all. I continued to be very active with housework, yard and had a garden, children and a husband to take care of, not to mention a lot of church duties. To my surprise I felt great and was starting to lose weight. On any high-protein or regular reducing diet I would lose weight and then after two weeks I couldn't stand it anymore, but with mild food it wasn't really hard not to cheat and want candy, etc.

Then, besides losing weight, my face cleared up and stayed that way except for two weeks when I was off of mild food at Christmas time, but as soon as I went on it again it cleared up. Also, within a few days of starting mild foods, I noticed my neck glands and throat felt a little sore. Not really hurting, just noticeably sore. The only illness I had had in the last six months was a sore throat. After Christmas when I started back on mild food after about a week, my nose started running a little. Then I had a real bad headache and realized I should be taking high doses of vitamin C so the mucus would dissolve and be able to get out easier. I did this and the next day my nose really started to run and mucus came out of my lungs also. These are the areas you can see in my eyes and eye slides that are weak and they are cleaning out and healing. Also, the parasite lines are going away in my eyes since taking black walnut.

Besides clearing up my skin, it's such a good texture and I have rosy cheeks for the first time since I was a little girl. Probably the best thing mild food and herbs have done for me, is something I didn't even realize until about a month ago, I don't have headaches anymore; I have always been headache prone. Let me get under a little pressure or have to hurry to get things done and I'll get a headache. It runs in my family. Anyway, one day I realized I hadn't had a headache in months. I am First Counselor in the Primary. I was in charge of the children's presentation at Sacrament meeting. Anyone who has had anything to do with these will know what a responsibility and challenge they are. I thought, "Well, this will really see what sort of shape I'm in." I went through several practices and the program, as worried and under stress as usual, but I didn't have headaches. This is possibly my strongest testimony that mild food and herbs work for me. There is no possible way I could've gone through these practices and that program without several headaches and lots of aspirin. I have always been that way before.

Carol Oster Miller

In giving my testimony of this program, I do so with much thankfulness. I have known for many years that we are, to the most part, what we eat. Through the years of soft drinks, french fries, and hamburgers, somewhere in my conscience, something warned me to take wiser care of my body, but I didn't listen until I needed to when much damage had already been done. Strangely enough, these problems didn't reveal themselves until I was married and expecting my first baby; when I had a nervous breakdown. This, of course, was brought on mainly by stress and a different way of living. My doctor treated me with tranquilizers and from that point on all things – all problems medically that I had – were attributed to nerves by the doctors. This stress started many other problems until after my fourth baby when I found I had osteoarthritis and ankylosing spondylitis, a hardening of the spine. I was told I would eventually need both hips replaced. There was no hope. Just years of suffering to look forward to. I felt absolutely defeated. Then through a good friend, I heard of the program of mild foods and herbs. Everything my friend told me seemed to ring logically true. I wanted to know more. LaDean Griffin, the lady my friend had learned the program from, was coming to give lectures, so I attended.

At first I couldn't believe what I was hearing. It was too simple. I prayed to know if it was true, and I received a beautiful, spiritual testimony of it. I live on the mild foods diet. I am taking herbs for my particular problems, and I personally believe they are helping me regain my health and strength. I know I am healing. It won't happen overnight, but I do know I will again have good health.

I've learned through personal experiences of friends that this program is true. I have seen it work. Through taking the herbs, black walnut, for instance, I can walk without pain, and before I was in constant pain – severe pain in my hips. Walking at times was the thing I had to mentally do to put one foot in front of the other and force myself to move. With black Walnut I can walk and not feel this pain. This program has brought me closer to my Father in Heaven. I have joy and a greater faith in tomorrow. I can weather the storms easier and rear my children in a quiet, peaceful home.

Simple truths have always been a stumbling block for people through the ages. I believe this program, simple as it is, to be part of the hidden treasures spoken of in the Latter-day Saint Word of Wisdom. God does provide if we are willing to search out the truth. For every problem there is an answer somewhere written, if we will search it out. For this I am truly grateful.

Dorothy Cook

when I started taking herbs I knew I would eventually start feeling better. What I didn't know was the full impact herbs would play in my own health and that of my entire family. I get so excited when I recall the change they came over me in just a few days of taking licorice root and a combination of gotu kola, ginseng and capsicum herbs. Absolutely a miracle! It is marvelous to wake up refreshed, full of energy, more tolerant of people and events, and a deep sense of well-being. Needless to say, I had no trouble getting my husband and children on herbs after they witnessed the change in me, and I'm happy to report the changes in them have been just as rewarding.

My husband and I are with each other constantly, as we own our own business and actually enjoy all this togetherness. Our children still tease and quarrel with each other, but with a much kinder tone of voice which in turn has stopped fights from erupting. In fact, our lives have reached the point where if one of us uses a tone of voice other than the nicest we have so quickly gotten used to, the comment made in response is, "Take your herbs!" We are all taking other herbs and food supplements now for certain health problems and weaknesses, there is no doubt in my mind that licorice root, gotu kola, ginseng and capsicum have made us feel so much better that we have the courage and desire to continue making the changes necessary in order to have more perfect health. Thanks be to God for

His wisdom in providing herbs for His children and for answering my prayers for better health and happiness for my family.

Overcomes tumors with herbs

I was sick most of my life, due to weakness, so when I found out about the herbs and supplements, I felt it was a blessing and an answer to my prayers. I've always wanted to help people and this was one way I could. Since I've been on the herbs, I've really noticed a change in my health. I had rheumatic fever as a child, three to five years old, and started developing arthritis, (rheumatoid) about 12 years of age. I had a weakness in my legs and my back (due to falls). Now, my hearts almost healed up, the weaknesses in my legs is almost gone and arthritis is diminishing.

I also to dig up quite a bit from 10 to 16 years of age; I was very nervous and had two ulcers during high school years. Half the time I chewed gum, I swallowed it. About two months ago I passed some gum. Last month I went on Doctor Jensen's garlic fast, and passed plastic. Since I have been on the herbs I have lost a fibroadenoma tumor. Doctors had decided it was a genetic defect and during removal of my first tumor, they saw my tissue was nodular. My second tumor caused them to conclude I would have more, but lucky for me, not cancerous tumors. I shrank that tumor with massive vitamin E supplements, then when I started taking herbs, I cut back and developed my third, which the combination CS shrank in two days.

My health has been improved in other ways too, and I believe I owe it all, first to the Lord and second and third to my loving parents, and my friend for being with me through this, and I know the best is yet to come.

I also lost approximately 10 unwanted pounds in six months with mild food diet, lecithin, and a combination of chickweed, licorice, saffron, gotu kola, mandrake, fennel, echinacea, and black walnut herbs, that helped my glands function properly.

Goiter disappears

I live in Bakersfield, California. I came into the knowledge of herbs some nine months ago. I have however been acquainted with the herbs for about 20 years and didn't realize it. In 1961 a surgeon told me my youngest daughter would have to have a goiter removed from her throat before she choked on it. I have baby pictures – she was born with it. Because of my diet – no eggs, greens, etc. on comfrey, kelp, and garlic tablets, I had her well in one year. I took her back to the doctor, he measured it, and it was gone and has never returned. I myself had a corn between my little toe for 20 years, it is now gone. According to iridology, my eyes were brown, now they are Hazel, no more gold tones in my brain area on the right side. I have a deformed rib, and injury, we found in my eye I never knew I had, that spot is almost gone. Also where I was kicked by a horse about 10 years ago (in the right ovary), also showed up in my eye with two spots, one is gone and the other going. I have had spotting in ovulation ever since the injury, now with the black cohosh, I do not spot anymore at all. I have had all the miserable things that women have to put up with at that time of the month, and I'm happy to say that I do not even know when the time is arriving (which can also be a problem).

My husband has not been able to sleep on his back since I married him because of a pain in his right shoulder and headaches. We gave him the gallbladder treatment and he passed 75 (or more) stones and some the size of my thumb. He sleeps like a baby now, no more pain in the shoulder. I had sinus also when I first got on to the herbs, I had more headaches than ever, and then I would drain and drain. Now I never have headaches and that is really great.

Earache and pneumonia

A friend of mine had a five-year-old boy who had a terrible earache. He'd had it for over a week without success from medication the doctor had given him. Out of desperation, my friend contacted me, and I told her about a garlic enema and vitamin C. She proceeded to give him 1000 mg of vitamin C every hour and painted his throat with iodine and glycerin every 15 minutes. Within two hours the swelling in his throat, which caused his earache, was gone and the pain was too. Within another hour, the child wanted to eat again. We gave him fruit for another 24 hours, with the vitamin C. By then the infection was gone and never returned. I have a daughter who has had pneumonia several times. It has never been an infectious type and had no fever with it, but still had all the other symptoms. The doctors never know what to do, as she does not respond to antibiotics. When I learned about the mild food diet, I put her on it. She has never had pneumonia again, however, if she gets too many concentrated foods, going off of the diet, she immediately starts with congestion, so she has to be very careful not to eat them too often or she could end up with any of the lung diseases. As for my own self, I had a period of time when I didn't feel good because of an adrenal problem. I acquired arthritis from this, so I now take licorice root, I feel better but I have a long way to go. My body was so weak that building with vitamin therapy was very essential to me. I now have about three weeks, pain-free and 10 bad days. I look forward to more good all the time.

Parts of a letter to Reverend Crosby

Dear Reverend Crosby:

I have just completed 10 days of taking your Herb Tea Formula. I cannot believe the results! This simple remedy of your herb formula accomplished what 35 specialists (including 15 at Mayo Clinic) were unable to do, and who could not even come close to it in the seven years I have been plagued with Systematic Lupus Erythematosus. The results from your seven-day fast, with juices and yogurt, was almost immediate. So much so, that I have not had an injection of gamma globulin for the last 10 days. I needed them every three or four days, using 45 CC's in June and July. The only problem I had was with the yogurt, as I am highly allergic to all dairy products.

Thank God I am now free of all headaches, which I had constantly. My illness began with a fever that lasted six weeks, around 101 to 102, and I am surprised that the drugs did not kill me. My hands were all covered with blisters for two years, and felt as though they were on fire. I would put them in ice cold water, to relieve the burning. It was always in the back of my mind to go on an herbalist, and now, you are my salvation. I have had so many injections, I am running out of skin.

The dear Lord heard my prayers and came to my aid when I received your formula. I still have a long way to go, but every day brings surprises and I am sure now that the formula will bring me the cure I have sought for so long.

Vanda Just

I have always had problems – health problems – all my life. Always infections. Gamma globulin has always been low, and my children have inherited these problems. Several places in my body were deformed from it. It little over a year ago a specialist told me that within the year I would not be pushing my own wheelchair. There was much pain with it, many problems, lots of medicine, gold shots, steroids, cortisones, on and on and on. But when the big expense came, it was with lupus. The arthritis had turned inward, and it acts the same as rheumatoid arthritis does, only it eats out the lining of your vital organs.

The doctors told me I was lucky last November because it was in the beginning stages, but it is terminal. I had been in so much pain. My skin was gray, my heart was bad, my eyes had sunken dark circles around them. It affected the family because everyone suffered. I had gotten so bad and filled with so much pain that one night in February, after my husband and I had gone to bed, I felt my heart stop. I felt my breathing stop, and my spirit came right out of my body. I can be up a dozen times with my children during the night and my husband never knows it, but something woke him up that night. He jumped and he grabbed for me and he called me because he knew something was drastically wrong. I couldn't hear him through my ears. I heard him through my spirit. It sounded as if it were 100 miles away. The pain came with pushing my spirit back into my body. I felt my breathing start. I felt my heart starts beating. I finally said to him, "I'm not going to make it." And he said, "you will now. You've got a pulse."

The next morning when we got up, I asked him if he had remembered this, and he said, "I know so much more than you. I know how close you came. I don't think you'll ever know." We decided to fast and pray because we knew healing was an answer. I had prayed for many years for healing of arthritis, but one night before February I was filled with the Holy Spirit and I felt the power of him in my hands. I touched the places that I was crippled and drew it out, but God did not seem to heal me of the lupus. There had to be a reason.

I still have arthritis, but I don't have the purple places, and it's very much controlled. But getting back to that time. We were talking, and the phone rang. A woman who owns a Health Food Store in Blackfoot called me. There had been a woman who walked into her store, she was from Logan, Utah and she was a friend and neighbor of LaDean Griffin. She saw the book on the counter and made a statement that her friend was going to be giving lectures in Rexburg, Idaho and then this friend told her about me and she said that LaDean Griffin had a friend that had lupus and that she had been learning about it and was getting good results, so please have me come. This friend called me and I knew instantly that this was the answer that God had given me. That was the answer to my prayer. I went up to Rexburg. I took the lectures and I quit all medications. I was on $250 worth of drugs a month, and they weren't helping me at all. They were just covering up the problem and there was still so much pain and agony and misery. In two months I have improved so greatly that our family attorney asked me for help. I referred him to LaDean's book and have helped many people this way. But what also brought it home was the fact that I've got a four-year-old child. All of his life he has had health problems like all the other children I've had. He's been on several Gamma globulin shots a month. He's had antibiotic shots, many of them a month. Bottles of antibiotics. Constant medicine, and he would lay there like a vegetable with no will to even get up and play, and I started him on liquid vitamins and minerals, high dosages of vitamin C, and that child has not had a shot or medication or anything in three months. He's a strong, healthy, normal child. I know his body has to clear out a lot of toxic waste, but he's well on the road to recovery. My 13-year-old several weeks ago had a very severe asthma attack, caused from being around horses. His fingernails and lips turned purple. His eyes rolled in the back of his head because of lack of oxygen. It's very frightening to use herbs, just herbs, when you're always used to the hospital and oxygen and you wonder, "Am I taking this child's life into my hands? What if I don't do it right?" It's frightening. For 36 hours we worked over that child, and he came out with flying colors. I've never seen him improve so quickly as he did on herbs of vitamin C. A year ago someone witnessed to me about herbs and I thought to myself, "Each to his own," and I didn't want to jeopardize my life by taking myself off of drugs and going on herbs, and yet, really, it was the other way around. I feel that the Bible proves that herbs are for the use of man for medicine, and I really feel this is a lesson that God wanted me to learn otherwise He would have healed me of the lupus and taken all the arthritis away instead of just the crippling. I feel it's going to be the answer and I really feel that if doctors would become more aware and use preventative medicines, such as herbs, in their practices that we wouldn't have so many problems. Many doctors are turning to this and it is proving to be very beneficial.

Shirley Yancey

I took the classes from LaDean Griffin about two years ago and have lived close to the laws of health, mild food and herbs to heal the body. Since I was a very nervous, depressed individual, living this program of health and reading the Scriptures pertaining to health convinced me, this is the way our Heavenly Father chose for His children to live because of its simplicity, not cutting into the body, and side effects of the drugs.

Taking these classes from LaDean Griffin has shown me this law. We live this, it gives us a freedom – freedom from the terror of dreaded disease. We have the assurance that something can be done and we, with the helpful prayers to our Father in Heaven who knows all laws, can free us from this bondage. As a mother, this has paid its dividends many times. Reading and studying, going to LaDean's classes and using herbs has brought our family through many illnesses and pain, but also as a mother it brings many burdens and heartaches. It's very difficult to try to convince members of a family to change their eating habits when we use the science of iridology and see that they have sick bodies but they are not willing to give up the traditional All-American hamburger, the hot dog and soda pop, to change from their meat, bread, sugar, and tacos to the use of fruits and vegetables. This is where the burden comes when those whom you love have used drugs for many years but their bodies are deteriorating with pain and cannot see the truthfulness of this law. These are the burdens that you have to bear. You also meet people who have been searching for this law who have gone the route of surgery and drugs and finally found this new Hope and are surprised by its simplicity. I must say that this has brought me much closer to my Heavenly Father. In order that we know the truthfulness of all things and feel His Spirit must guide us whenever we change our lives for improvement we need His help. I've called on Him many times and felt of His direction. I feel fortunate that over two years ago I went to LaDean Griffin's classes and could partake of her many, many years of study and research, that my health can be changed. I feel fortunate also for this blessing to me that I can help others and this law will bless their lives.

Shirley Rawlings

I went to LaDean's classes for three days, the next day my father came over. He had had a real critical accident in a saw, with his hand, and he almost lost his little finger on his right hand. It had cut him in several places. When he came to my home, it was just heavily invaded with infection, and it was brilliant, Scarlet red. Immediately I saw the infection, and so I decided that it needed to be soaked and that there must be an herb that would draw this out so I mixed the paste of Lobelia with vitamin E oil. I put the paste on his finger, and then we put just a small bandage around it so that the air was still circulate. It hadn't been on his hand very long and he looked at me and he said, "Boy, that is really potent salve that you put on my finger. I can feel it begin to draw." Well, we kept this on for three days, and we kept soaking it three times a day and put the Lobelia on three times a day. By the next Monday we took the Lobelia off and just started putting goldenseal and myrrh mixed with vitamin E oil on it. About a week and a half later, it was healed and starting to close. The infection is all gone, and we're just keeping vitamin E oil on it to keep it from scarring.

My little boy had a wart on his finger, and since I knew that the Lobelia would pull things, I decided to put it on to see if I could pull a wart. After I put it on the first night, well, the next morning you can see the little roots starting to pull up and you can see the roots come off and within three days the work came off.

Peggy Burnshaw

Lavon: "When did you first hear about the mild food and the herbs?"

Peggy: "When Sister Griffin came last August."

Lavon: "Did you stay on the mild food after that?"

Peggy: "Yes, in fact I stayed on it for 21 days without stopping. I didn't snitch once. I was so proud of myself. I felt better than I've ever felt. In fact, I'd just had my baby. She was about three months old. I had a terrible pregnancy. My nose was red the whole time. My nose and my face were red and my back was always breaking out and things like that. I couldn't understand that, and I felt terrible, always tired. I was eating liver until it came out my ears. After I started on the diet, about three days afterwards, my nose completely cleared up, and went to the normal color of my face. I was eating a lot of avocados – it was that time of year, my skin turned really nice. In fact I felt really good. I must not have been very weak because I didn't have many bad days at all. In fact, sometimes I felt like I could just fly. It just felt so good."

Lavon: "Did you take any herbs at all?"

Peggy: "No, when we first heard it, I was nursing the baby and you know, all the propaganda that goes around, what you need to nurse your baby, this and that, and I was just so concerned about losing my milk, and so when I went on mild foods, I figured I'd better not go on anything stronger, so I didn't go on CS or anything like that for a long time and then it was about a month before I got going on licorice. You know, it takes all this stuff a while to sink in until you can understand it, and so we didn't do very much of that, but with my baby I took a lot of vitamin C when her nose was running and that really helped her and I gave her several enemas, and that would clear her fever up just really fast. My husband went hunting and they ate meat and another things after he been on mild foods for a long time and he was really sick. Anyway, his eyes are bad, and when he got sick, everyone said, and he said, "Oh, I know it's the meat. That is what's done it." Mel's kind of crazy anyway. They got Aspen bark and made a tea of it, and it cleared everything right up. They all said it's because it would taste so horrible it would cure anything. I've been taking licorice now really a lot and the CS, my baby's eyes are just really changing, and they were really horrible for a little baby. It scared me to death, but not anymore, you know. She'd have probably got really sick very young. Her eyes were almost a brown-red color, and now I think they're going to be gray and there is really a lot that has cleared out. My husband's eyes have changed and my eyes are also changing.

I haven't stayed on the diet, like a Christmas time, we blew it, and ever since then it's been like a week on and three days off and a week on and a week off. But always our diets have improved just enormously. And so, from our eyes, there's a difference. I have taken a lot of herbal pumpkin and lately a lot of iodine. Lately, really strong on things, so I'm sort of anxious to tell."

Lavon: "Are your eyes fading off?"
Peggy: "Yes, I'm anxious to see my next pictures. My husband's eyes have changed a lot, and he's taken the black walnut. We've taken a lot of it. Black Walnut and CS. Lately I think my vitality is up because I have a white tongue, so as long as my tongue's white, I don't worry."

In order to eliminate we have to have vitality and we know when the tongue whitens, the elimination is beginning to happen.

Melva Splenik

I started on this program in August, and at this time I started on the mild food diet and I went on it up until November. I gained 40 pounds on the mild food diet and that was a real shock to me. But what happened was, I filled with fluid, then my kidney stopped functioning. In December I saw your mother, LaDean. She taught me a whole new idea – mild foods and herbs. I set myself up on a program. The kidneys started functioning again, but I was still retaining water, and I know that I am a hyperglycemic. I've learned this, and I have heart trouble. Before this particular time I had been on heart medication for a good five years. I went off my heart medication and all drugs completely. I wasn't taking any after that at all. And I had somewhere from 6 to 8 spells with my heart, and I wasn't familiar with the Hawthorn berries. The only thing I really was aware of was how well cayenne worked, so I got on cayenne and started taking three capsules a day. Whenever I'd have a spell, I'd take 2 teaspoons in water, and it worked just like nitroglycerin and stopped the spell instantly. This was quite an experience.

Lynn: "Did you stay on the mild food diet strictly?"

Melva: "I did up until about December when I gained all this weight, then I got to panicking and thinking and reading and I studied on hyperglycemia, and I thought, boy, I'm not doing the right thing, and I got to panicking because I was getting so big. So I thought I'd better add a little protein back into my diet, and this is what I started doing. I started back on protein. Well, first I started with taking yeast. I found that eating meat, after that length of time, I got sick, and it bothered me, so I started taking some yeast. In about the middle of January, I had a cleanse, a really big cleanse, and I passed a worm, we decided, that was 6 inches long. We looked at it, and we decided – we didn't know what kind it was – but we knew that it was of the worm family. You could see it."

So I stayed on this protein and I started losing a little bit of the fluid, and now I started back on the diet again. I've lost 10 pounds since I came on the diet. But the thing I'm not sure about is, I don't know whether I have Addison's disease or not. I might be in the further state, but I don't know. I've been taking four capsules of licorice a day, and I take vitamin E. I also take a combination of Hawthorn berries and capsicum, and I've noticed – we talked about it in class today – that if you have bumps on your thumps in your heart and I've noticed since the time that I went on this that mine has flattened out and I no longer have these bumps, so I know that the heart has improved. I no longer have the heart spells that I was having.

I can see a definite change in my eyes. I've noticed that the colon has cleaned up considerably. My nerve rings were really bad. They have really lightened and phased, a great deal. The parasite lines have phased away, and there is a definite change in the thyroid. I know that my thyroid glands are still bad, because I can feel them. They hurt at times, and I can see it in my eyes, but it's starting to phase off, too. Possibly, when I reach that certain point, I expect to lose some of this fluid I'm still retaining. I think it's because all the glands are out of balance and aren't working together. I might add, that I decided that I went into the cleanse too quick, because I went mostly on fruit, and a person that's been sick for years – in fact for 10 years I've been really chronically sick. My body was not strong enough to go into this cleanse, and so it threw me in so fast when I started on fruit that I decided this is what stopped the function of the kidneys, and I just plain got sick. The kidneys had stopped for a good eight hours, and I was administered to and my name was turned in to the temple at this particular time. My kidneys stopped in the morning, and it was midnight that night that they started functioning again they've never quit completely since, but they still are not working completely right. One other thing I might add that I have been doing for kidneys. I've been drinking 2 cups of sagebrush tea and this is really been helping to keep my kidneys moving.

Lorna Stratinger

My husband and my little boy and I have been on the mild food diet for about six months. At first we went on a lot of potatoes because we were really hungry, but we never felt so good in all our lives. And at first we were really, really nervous because I am sure we were cleansing and I have always been a nervous person. In fact, I was on tranquilizers in high school. I'd lay in bed and shake and throw up my food. I couldn't sleep, and things were really bad. Now I sleep like a rock and take lots of vitamin B and calcium and licorice root. I feel like I've learned something new in the last classes because I quit taking licorice root and now I find that I'm hyperglycemic, and I thought it was hypo with the symptoms. Now I take goldenseal – one goldenseal to every two licorice in the morning, and I do it again at night. Then I take saffron to utilize my fruit, and I can see that that's really helped me because I haven't been able to utilize my fruit before. My complexion is cleared up. I feel so good, and I hope I don't lose any more weight. I feel good, and I have energy. I feel like I want to get up in the morning instead of laying in bed, and that's just occurred in the last two weeks.

My husband does a 1000 push-ups a day and he boxes and his eyes are full of white. He's so strict he never goes off the mild food diet. He knows that – we feel that this is a celestial law and will be living this way someday, so we want to try to clean our bodies up and learn about herbs so that we can help others who may not be able to learn about this. The time's coming when they'll need help and when they're sick and can't get doctors.

Lavon: "Have you noticed a change in your eyes?"
Lorna: "Yes, I have a really, really bad colon, and it makes lots of jigs and jags and it was black, destroyed tissue there and destroyed tissue in my ovary area, that's why am not pregnant. That's the reason I'm taking the formula, and I'm taking it twice a day and I can see white in quite a few areas of my eyes now."

Geraldine Cook

I have had severe migraine headaches for some 35 years of my life. I have tried doctors, medication. The winter of 1975 I spent in Mesa, Arizona and I went to Phoenix to three headache specialists. They took the brainwave. They took the brain scan, and they put me in the hospital for two days, and they didn't find anything; so, when I came home my sister told me about this program. I got a letter from a doctor at Stanford University saying that they wanted me there on the sixth of May for one more test, and this was after LaDean's first-class. I was so impressed, that I wrote a letter and told the doctor, "I'm tired of drugs, I'm tired of getting nowhere. I have found the answer." So immediately I went to the health store, got the herbs that she told us about, CS, and I'm on the lower bowel, but there's another for headache.

Lavon: "A combination of valerian root, wild lettuce and capsicum?"

Geraldine: "Yes, and no headaches. They're going," so I told him "I'm going to do it naturally this time because at last I had found the answer, so I wouldn't be there." So, maybe they'll look into it and see that this is the only way. I went on mild food. I had my husband on mild foods. He was treated in Arizona, also, for one month, four days a week, for emphysema.

Lavon: "How's he doing?"
Geraldine: "Well, I've got him on this program, off the drugs, onto the lung herbs and also the Hawthorn Berry for his heart, and were on the juices. We went over and bought a juicer, so it's changed both of our lives, but I thought I was doomed to have these migraine headaches, and I'm engaged in the field of genealogical work, and I wanted so bad to get back to it and now I feel the Lord has helped me to get here to this class."

Gloria G. Lowry

in 1960 in the late fall I became aware that there was something very wrong. I went to my doctor, and I said, "There is something very, very wrong with me, and I'm not really sure what it is," and he gave me a rather perfunctory examination, and said, "Oh, all you need is for spring to come."

I didn't really believe it, but I accepted it. In April when we returned from Conference I went back to him, after having had a very dreadful experience with extreme nervousness, tearfulness, and feelings of hostility, and I went back to him and he said, "You have a double goiter." I had a hyperactive thyroid gland and my eyes were already bulging. It took him until July to build me up to the point where they dared to perform surgery.

During this time I lost a great deal of weight, became very, very nervous and began to experience and manifest symptoms of neurosis, and so after the surgery he said he would release me in the care of a psychiatrist, and he did. The psychiatrist was just opening his practice and was trying to make a name for himself and I suppose, really, I became a kind of guinea pig.

They began to treat me in the traditional way with psychotherapy and drugs. I alternated between depression and rebellion, and as I would begin to rebuild against the treatment he would raise the level of medication, and I stayed with this man for about nine years, during which time we paid him $20,000 in drugs and medical costs, and he told me that I was schizophrenic and continued to adjust the medication to try to help me maintain some level of stability because my body could not handle these things. It was a very difficult situation, and I became depressed and suicidal on two or three occasions and he put me into a private mental hospital and treated me with shock treatments and medication. It was a very difficult experience. I've had 21 shock treatments. Eventually, we went to Washington, DC on a sabbatical leave. He told me that I would always have to take therapy and that I would have to have periodic shock treatments throughout the rest of my life. When we went to Washington, DC, I realized that I did not need to see this man every week or every two weeks as he had led me to believe, and although I was functioning on a relatively low efficiency level, I was functioning. While I was in Washington, I had periods of dizziness and a great craving for sugar and candy, and I tried all these years to live the kind of life I had been used to living – creative and busy and active, and it was very, very difficult under that kind of medication, as I slept a good deal of the time. My children, when they were very young, thought that I was a witch. So, while I was in Washington I craved sugar, I remember on one occasion I went to a candy store and bought a 2 pound box of peanut brittle and ate it in one sitting, and I continued to indulge myself in sugar because I was so weak, and I thought I was taking a high energy boost.

On Mother's Day that year I took the children out to dinner. My husband was out west on business. We had a lovely dinner and dessert, and then we went back to sacrament meeting. Following sacrament meeting, I became quite dizzy and faint feeling, and I said to the girls, "We must leave." I made it just barely out of the chapel into the foyer and passed out, so they put me into the hospital, and the doctor who had been treating me – I found a doctor when we went to Washington to supervise the medication which I was taking – was called when I went into the hospital, and he didn't even speak to me. I was dizzy. He said, "What are you doing in here?", and I said, "Well,

I passed out in church," and that was last word he spoke. He did not examine me. He did not touch me. He did not do anything at all, just wrote on his pad of paper and then released me. And I was extremely dizzy and very, very ill.

My neighbor was extremely upset. I was having hearing problems. I couldn't hear the doorbell ring, and there was noise in my ears, and so she called her doctor and arranged for a specialist to see me and he said, "They should never have released you from the hospital," and they put me back in. They did a blood sugar test. An internist came and did a blood sugar test, and he said, "Your body doesn't seem to handle carbohydrates well," and I said, "Does that mean I have diabetes?" And he said, "No, you are not a true hypoglycemic, either, but I would suggest that when you return home you go to an internist and have this checked out." Well, I thought, you know, that if I didn't have diabetes and I couldn't handle carbohydrate and I was gaining weight so rapidly that I was just going to get big and fat if I didn't stop eating candy, but I couldn't seem to.

During the years under the psychotherapy the psychiatrist felt that it would be a tragedy if I were to have another child, and he insisted on putting me on the birth control pill, and I gained 50 pounds in the year. I insisted on going off the pill. When you're under this kind of medication, you really do not have control. You think and you have desires, but you are not able to express them and certainly not able to assert yourself against a powerful personality, and this was the situation in which I found myself. So, when we returned to Michigan I went back to the psychiatrist, and I said, "I want to discontinue treatment," I said, "I will take the medication, but I want to discontinue treatment." He said, "No, you must always have someone to supervise," and I said, "Well, all I really need is a chemist," and he smiled and said, "Well, I'll be your chemist." Well, I didn't want him to be my chemist. I didn't want any further to do with him, but I believed that I would always have to take Thorazine, and so I agreed then to continue the treatments, so that I would have another prescription written. He wrote them only for the period of time between visits, and this was going to be a once a month checkup. So he gave me a prescription for Thorazine that would last a month.

Then, when I got home I called and told him that I would discontinue treatment, and he sent a real scare letter to my husband.

Now, over all this time he was treating me, I was on various levels of medication. For a period of years I was on 350 to 375 mg of Thorazine a day, and then when I became depressed on that, he then gave me a reduced dosage and an antidepressant, so in effect I was on an upper and a downer, as the young people today say. Then, I came west with this one month of medication. I had great fear in my heart because I really believed I had to have it. And I didn't have a doctor. I talked to my cousin, who is a medical doctor and he said, "There's nothing schizoid about you. There never has been." And he said, "If you really want a psychiatrist, find someone else. Don't take that kind of a diagnosis from any one man." So, I went back home, and I wanted desperately to get off the medication, so I went to a general practitioner, whom I had not met. And he said, "I do not understand this drug, and I would be reluctant to take you off of it." He recommended another psychiatrist in town. Now, he took me off the drug immediately. He didn't work me off from it at all, he just said, "Stop taking it." At that time I must've been taking, perhaps 175 mg of Thorazine and I don't know what the other one was, the upper. But, I had tremendous withdrawal symptoms. He continued to check me and after three weeks, he said to me, "I wish that we had more people in the world with your maturity and with your stability, it's interesting to me that the other psychiatrist was not able to reprogram your mind," and I said, "Well, there were two things going for me, I have a very strong spirit and the Lord was on my side."

And the Lord continued to be on my side, but I was very frightened because I was alone and, as I would go to a doctor for help, they would want to know, what is it that's wrong, and as soon as they would find out that I'd been under psychiatric care, they would label me as neurotic, and if they couldn't determine what was wrong with me, it had to be in my mind, and it didn't really matter what the complaint was, it had to be in my mind. This attitude carried over to other members of my family. It was a very frustrating experience. So, I tried to live with it. I was very, very weak. I had periods of extreme weakness and faintness. For about a year I tried to take care of my home and my responsibilities. When the weakness would become too great I would lie on the floor till I could get up and do a few more things, and then I'd have to lie down again. But I continued to fight to maintain some normal life.

Through all of this my wonderful, wonderful husband was a tower of strength. Extremely frustrated. He had sought the best medical help he knew. He simply did not know what to do. He did all they could, having faith that he was doing all he could do and trusting those who were treating me. But the Lord was really watching over us and all these years my name was in the temple and many people prayed for me and encouraged me by helping me to continue to struggle. A friend then called me. I had become ill again after I had gotten off the Thorazine and away from the second psychiatrist. He saw no need to continue treatment. And I was just so very, very weak, and I felt as though I had the flu. I went into the doctor, and he tested me. He gave me a blood test, and he said, "You appear to have a virus. I'd like you to go home and take aspirin and go to bed," which I did for two weeks, and I didn't feel any better, so I went back, he did another blood test, and he said, "This is extremely interesting. You're white count is exactly where it was." He said, "These tests were done by two different technicians and its extremely unusual. I would like you to go home and take aspirin and go to bed." So, I did, but you can't really stay in bed when you have a family and you have a life to live, and I began to try to function. Then, I was visiting a friend, and I passed out. We were practicing a musical number we were going to do in church when I passed out. They took me to an osteopathic hospital, and they did many, many tests, I was there for two weeks, and as I now realize, I must've been going out – in and out of insulin shock because I was not able to eat, and so I was fasting. Well, now that I'm on mild foods, I also realize that there were many poisons already out into my system and moving, and they didn't understand it, and I certainly didn't understand it, they would give me additional medication, and it was really a very hellious time.

During that period of time, I had a woman come into my room to be a roommate who had been in great pain and had not been able to sleep for a week, and she was such a brave little thing, and didn't complain at all. I couldn't bear to see her in that kind of agony and I just asked the Lord to bless her that she would be able to rest. I continued to pray and continued to watch her. I raised up on my elbow and stayed on my elbow, leaning up, as long as I possibly could, concentrating on her and praying that the Lord would grant her some rest. She dropped off to sleep and remained sleeping till I was too weak to continue and dropped off myself. She said, "That was almost a miracle, I haven't slept for such a long time." I then gained a testimony that the Lord can heal and the thing that we are taught, that faith can heal was a valid thing, and it moved beyond faith, but to an absolute knowledge that when we ask, having faith, we will be given the answer. I asked, having faith, for myself and I didn't seem to have the answer that instantaneously, and it was sobering and it was a little frustrating. I decided that for some reason the Lord didn't want to reach down and touch me and make me well, that I needed to find solutions to the problem. And I continued in this manner.

I spent two years – two summers – during the past three or four years in Salt Lake City and Provo undergoing many, many, tests under the care of my dear cousin who loves me dearly and would move heaven or hell to help me, and I realize that. They really and truly could not pinpoint exactly what was going on. I have a borderline hypoglycemia. The manifestation was too dramatic, and they really felt that much of this was in my mind. At one point, after I had been two or three weeks in the hospital, I was released, I was in great pain, and they didn't know what was wrong, I became very, very depressed. I had been taking a mild sedative because I was not able to sleep, and he felt I needed rest and apparently it built up in my body.

I got up one morning at mother's house, and I said, "I'm going for a walk," and she said, "All right, but your weak. You've been in the hospital for a couple of weeks, so be careful. Don't go too far." So, I said, "I won't." I had an ice pick in my hand and I walked as far as I can walk in a numb, disorganized fashion, as far as I could walk down into a cornfield and fell and lay there trying to get the courage to stab myself. But they had missed me and were praying for me and the Lord was watching over me, and I did not do this horrible thing which, of course I did not want to do and would not even have considered had it not been for the drugs in my system. And I came to, after several hours of sleeping and waking and sleeping and waking in this cornfield, and dragged myself to the road and a young man picked me up and put me in the car and took me to the hospital. I was deeply depressed and I refused any kind of medication, and I refused any kind of food and, of course, they can't give it to you if you refuse it now. In years past they could.

Paul became deeply frustrated. He didn't know what to do, and he said, "If we can't get her to eat or to accept help, I'll have no alternative but to put her in the psychiatric ward at the University. The poor little darling has given up hope." My husband called. He, of course, was with the children in Michigan, and he called and he tried to encourage me, and he began to give me a blessing and to pray for me over the telephone, and I hung up. And I attempted suicide that night. I had a glass of water, and I was going to break it and they could sense that and they kept a nurse in the room all evening and I don't really know what happened, but something did, and I changed my mind and permitted them to give me medication and they brought me out of it. But, unfortunately, it was another antidepressant and it only compounded the problem. It was a very, very difficult struggle to continue to strive, continue to stay faithful, continue to have hope, to continue to pray, and to continue to try to function on a meaningful level, but I was able to and I'm very grateful.

The following year I made the acquaintance of a man who uses hypnotherapy, and he, through this technique, helped me to understand my feelings toward the psychiatrist and the understanding that I was not a total loss, and he planted again within my heart real hope and faith. This man, unfortunately, has been led astray. At that point in time he had been led astray by the religions of the East, and many of the things that he told me I countered with my own deep faith and would not accept even in hypnosis. Eventually, I came to the point where I could no longer use hypnosis, and I feel that the Lord blessed me there. He permitted me to have enough of the experience to free myself so that I could move on, and then He removed me from danger. I have a great testimony in the love and compassion and patience of the Lord in spite of the fact that we are so stupid and so stubborn.

I began to have increasing weak spells, falling into a gray-out, not a total blackout, but a gray-out experience where I can hear things going on about me, but I could not respond, and this continued for about a year, and I never knew when I left home whether I would get back or not, whether I would end up in the hospital or just what would happen, and we lived in a kind of a low anxiety. But you can't really just give up and lie on the bed. I guess you can, but I'm not that kind of person, and so early last spring I was shopping, and I felt ill. The doctor told me to carry candy with me, and when I felt ill eat candy or sugar. It was as though a switch had flicked in my brain somehow in my head. It was almost a physical thing, and then I would sink in varying degrees of rapidity into this gray-out, and I ate the sugar. I was in a large discount store and I tried to make my way to the front, and I just barely got there, then I passed out and they put me in the hospital. I was there for a week and they did tests. There were two internists who came in, new doctors who did not know that I had a "psychiatric problem". Two internists came in to treat me one of whom believed that I had a real problem and the other thought I was craving attention. Little did he know, because I had all the love and attention any human being could want, and many rich blessings of which I was fully aware. I was in the hospital for a week, and during that time I would go into the insulin shock and they really and truly did not understand what was happening. At one point, when I went into the shock, they had been treating me with orange juice and sugar and I told the nurse – I felt this happen and I said, "I must have some juice and sugar," and she said, "All right," but she didn't come. She was busy with other things, and she didn't come, when she came I was semi-conscious. So, she attempted to feed it to me with a syringe orally and I nearly choked, I suppose. It was rather ghastly. So, they called for a blood sugar test. Well, I have had sufficient orange juice and sugar that the level in the test was in a reasonable low range of normal, because I was only semi-conscious. I heard the two technicians say, "She's just pulling a bluff. This is not a real comatose situation".

As I came out of it – and I do tend to come out of it, not rapidly and not to a very high level – sugar apparently had some effect – and I came out of it and remembered and realized what had been said, and I called the nurse and I asked to see the head nurse. They came and I said, "I have been through hell. Please do not put me back in." And the head nurse apologized and said that conversation ought never to have taken place." I said, "But, it did, and I do not want it on my record. I have been through hell. Please don't put me back in."

After period of time I was released. I was home for just a week again to the store and this time I had my daughter with me because I was afraid to go alone. It takes a while to get up your courage again. My daughter was 13, and I felt this happened to me, and I said, "I'm going to be ill, Amanda. Go call daddy." We happened to be standing by a candy counter, and I remembered that the doctor said that chocolate candy would probably pull me out of it more rapidly than sugar cubes. So, I reached over and picked up a package of chocolate bars, but could not think how to open it. I could not remember. I could not function enough to open it. A couple came by, I remember them vaguely, an older couple, and he said to me, "Are you ill?" And I said, "Yes." He said, "Do you have a sugar problem?" And I said, "yes." And he unwrapped the candy bar, but by then I was too weak to chew it and they took me into the back room and waited for my husband. They were not able to revive me, so they put me in an ambulance and took me to the hospital. My husband, of course, followed in the car after having taken the children home. During that interval, when I was in the emergency room, I began to have severe tremors and the doctor in charge thought that I was having a grand mal attack and he screamed that he wanted Dilantin, and they gave me a heavy dose of Dilantin and, of course I was no epileptic so it did not have any positive effect. After they gave me the dilantin and it didn't bring me out of this tremor and out of the problem I was having, they decided to keep me and do some tests and, of course, I had already had every test in the book about 60 times, but this doctor didn't know it; so, I went upstairs, and because it seemed to be a brain problem, they put me into the ward where they have people who have had strokes, and things like this. They continued to give me Dilantin, and I was allergic to it. I broke out in a rash, and they thought I had measles, but instead of discontinuing the Dilantin because the tremors were continuing to come, the seizures, they gave me Benadryl to correct the allergic reaction, but I'm not able to handle antihistamine drugs and it only compounded it and I became anxious and then depressed and upset and so they gave me a tranquilizer to counter that reaction and after three weeks time and under these heavy medications it was an extremely difficult situation, and I became very frightened. They finally decided they could do no more, that I would be as well off at home, and I was released.

I decided that I had had all I could cope with, that I did not know what else to do. I had put my faith in the doctors. I had done diligently all that they had asked me to do, and I had continued to pray for guidance. But when I was released from the hospital in this dreadful state, I made a covenant with the Lord that if He would help me to get well I would not put another chemical into my body, and I have honored that and it has been very difficult to be in pain and have these situations occur and not to have medicine as I had been led to believe I needed to have. I've found that I've got along just as well, if not better, without it. I continued to have these blacking out spills. Then I went to the Word of Wisdom and decided that I would learn to live the way the Lord wanted me to, because I had long since realized that it's what you put into your body that creates or destroys good health.

While I was in the hospital with the Dilantin and all the other horrors, a young friend from our ward came to me and said, "Sister Lowry, you've helped me and I have a book that I think might be helpful to you," and it was Sister Griffin's book. Now, I was under heavy medication and I flipped through it and I read such things as herbs and things and I thought, "Oh, dear, here's another kooky health-food book," and I said, "I appreciate your bringing it, but I really have not been much of a health-food person." Oh, she said, "That's fine," and she left, and then I thought, "How ungracious of me to have been, not even to look at it," so I called her and I said, "I apologize. I really would like to look at the book," and so she ordered one for me. As I read it again I thought, "This is a lot of garbage." I guess I just wasn't humble enough.

This was a year ago. Over this past year, I have read the Word of Wisdom and prayed a great deal. I have read everything I can find on nutrition, and many new studies, of course, have been done concerning the addition of bulk and the effectiveness of vitamin C in dissolving cholesterol. I read John A. Widtsoe's Word of Wisdom, and I began to feel that I was on the right track, that I really needed the right kind of food.

It began about a year and half ago, and at that time I had gone out to eat at a restaurant that weekend and about three days later I became very ill with something that seemed like salmonella only far worse. I had sort of a locked jaw where I couldn't open my mouth and some shaking chills and diarrhea. Anyway, I was very, very ill for about four days. Finally, I talked to a doctor on the phone and he prescribed Lomotil and tetracycline, which at that time I took. I didn't get better, I just kept with the shaking chills and the diarrhea. In fact, even the American Medical Association has come out and said Lomotil should never be used, and it turned out later that I had para-typhoid fever which you would never use a strong anti-diarrheal for because it just backs it up in your system and that's what happened. It went all through my body, and into my lymph system and everything.

Until that time I had always felt pretty well all my life. The only thing that I can remember happening was about five years previous I developed sort of a coated geographic tongue that never disappeared. I was sick all the time, yet I didn't feel sick, and I'd asked various doctors about it, they would say, "Oh, it's nothing, nothing, it doesn't mean anything," and so I just kind of passed it off. Well, then, with this disease or whatever it was, I couldn't get out of bed, except to go to the bathroom, and I just never got better. I just stayed profoundly weak – most profound weakness – and I'd shake practically all night, and I'd just pile on the blankets. I ran a fever and it would never go away. I had it for five months with no help. I'd go to various doctors and they do all these tests. Then finally I wound up in the hospital, and they ran all these tests and didn't find anything, and so, finally I made an appointment with a specialist, one of the doctors did. He said, "It acts sort of like parasites, but we can't find them." Then this doctor sent me to the University of Utah Medical Center and the gastrointestinal specialists, because this doctor in Provo thought that it must have something to do with that, because I had diarrhea and everything. Then he checked me and he said that he strongly suspected that it was regional enteritis which was too bad, that it was incurable, and that the only way to test it was to open me up and go in and cut me open and find out, because there's no way to find it except by the symptoms, and my symptoms were classic symptoms of regional enteritis. He didn't recommend cutting me open because there was nothing they could do for it anyway, and so – the symptoms are the fever and profound weakness. The only way they try to take care of it is, they keep taking out part of the intestine and the colon to kind of halt it a little bit to try to give a remission to the disease, and it doesn't work very well at all. It's not a cure.

Just about two weeks before this I was in desperation and I got in the car one day and I decided, "I've got to find the answer," and, of course, I had prayed diligently all this time and I can remember saying, "If I don't care where the answer comes from; I'm willing to do anything, you know, to get the answer," and so I got in the car, my husband said he would keep the children. I just drove, and I went over to a clinic – it was some baby doctor clinic. It wasn't even my baby doctor, and I went in there and a nurse took me by the hand. She said, "Come here and talk to this doctor about your problem." And I went in there and he told me, "You know I have seen cases of salmonella in children that they couldn't even find the parasite or anything," but he knew it was there, whether their tests found anything or not. He said he's sure because he could give the drugs that they give for it and alleviate the problem. So then he took me by my hand and said, "Just remember, the medical profession does not know everything." This hit me just like a light bulb, and so I got in the car and I started driving. It was the strangest thing. And someone had told me before that there was an herb shop near my home and I went to this herb shop and walked in the door and just said. "I have been ill and I just don't know really what to do." She sold me some herbs, I think it was red Clover Blossom combination and some for nerves because by then I had never been in such a state. I was just a nervous wreck because I couldn't take care of my family. I had none of my family members here to help me, so I just didn't know what I was going to do. These herbs were teas, some herb teas. I started using them and I didn't really see any results. For one thing I was eating exactly the way I had before. I wasn't doing anything about diets. Nothing about diet, so I continued the same. I grew up in Virginia where you eat a lot of pork and you eat a lot of meat and you eat a lot of greasy foods.

My parents came to help me. My father and mother were there for two weeks, and I didn't get any better. I had started on these teas and my father and mother said, "This just can't go on." I had already had a blessing at the first of the disease, but my dad said, "We'll have to give you a blessing," so my father-in-law and my father blessed me, and the next morning I went upstairs. I never passed anything strange in my stool before, but that morning and that whole day I passed nothing but white mucus after that blessing and so I knew that there was an answer. Even though I kind of realized I wasn't going to be cured, you know, overnight or I didn't have the faith, I don't know what but I knew, there was something in there. You know, the doctors kept saying there's nothing in there, nothing in there, and when I asked the doctor in Salt Lake about it he said, "Well, we don't know what causes it. We don't know what it is. We don't have any idea, and there's no way to get rid of it." But Bill and I saw all this mucus coming out. You don't really pass all that much with the disease but you do pass mucus with it occasionally, but not this great. In fact, that whole day, that was all I passed. That was sort of an answer, so I knew there was an answer.

I went down to another health food store and there was a sign up that said "Iridology", and of course, I was intrigued by that. I decided to take this class. I could hardly get out of bed to go to LaDean's class.

Lavon: "Then you heard about her lectures?"
Gloria: "Yes. I read it on the sign. Iridology class, by LaDean. I went to her class. I could see the doctor was wrong, that I could probably cure this incurable disease."

Lavon: "What was your feeling when you heard LaDean?"
Gloria: "Oh, well I came home and I can remember telling my husband that night – so weak, "You know, there's very few times in my life I've really felt that the person that was talking to me was inspired and I was getting just about nothing but the truth, you know, and this occurred tonight."

Lavon: "This is what you prayed for?
Gloria: "Oh, yes, I know it's an answer to my prayer, that I was led, step-by-step to her. So, I knew it was the answer. I knew I had a long way to go, but I was going to try it. Then I started the mild food diet.

Lavon: "You bought her book, I guess?"

Gloria: "I bought her book and studied it cover to cover and started taking the CS and the herbal pumpkin and then I started the strangest thing, too. I took the fig formula that was the first herb I really took. I hadn't started the other one, and I couldn't believe it. Because of her book and changing the diet – you see, the other herbs didn't do much, when I was taking those teas I didn't really notice them, but when I started the diet and took herbs – Wow! My nose started immediately cleaning. Well, in fact the first day I ate nothing but fruit. That was probably a mistake because I was so weak."

Lavon: "Cleansing fast?"

Gloria: "Yes, well, I haven't really been that sick. What happened was that my nose just drained and my eyes and my neck hurt right where my lymph glands are and I wasn't expecting this, and it took me another class of LaDean's to realize – to know what to expect. A couple of days passed and then it would hurt in my lymph glands and my arms."

Lavon: "You told me you had lumps under your arms?"

Gloria: "Well, it kind of swelled up a little bit and then it would hurt and, of course, some of these things are sort of frightening because I'm new at this, but I still realized that I had been led to this answer. I tried to keep my cool. So, then I stayed on it exactly 3 months. In fact I just couldn't believe it. I got really, really sick. It was the first time I got really sick. But the interesting thing, the doctor told me this fever would not go away, that I'd just keep it. After being on this diet for two weeks the fever was gone from this disease, so that was something. In three months I had this big crisis, which I just couldn't believe. I passed nothing but mucus and ropes of mucus – black, dark brown and black, that color, you know, poisonous. It wasn't the white that I'd had before, that I'd had that one time when I had the blessing. I guess – I don't know what the black means compared to the white. Maybe it's digging deeper, but anyway, I was very sick. I was only sick for 2 1/2 days. It was just amazing. I couldn't believe I can be that sick for that short period of time and then get better."

Lavon: "You must have passed that poison out in that short period of time?"

Gloria: "Yes, and then it left and then I was better than I was before. I went back to Virginia and stayed on the diet, I'm sure there were some things that were in the foods, I know that mother would occasionally slip butter into the peas and things like that, but I stayed on the fruits and vegetables and then four months later, I had another healing crisis. I can remember, at the fourth month. I hadn't eaten for 2 1/2 days, and yet I went in and pass this thing at least a foot and a half long of rope of just straw. It was just hard. What it was well, it reminded me of when you're clearing a drain and it's gotten all stopped up and it's been stopped up for a week or something – a month – and you know how it's kind of slimy and black all up in the drain. I passed so much that I'm sure it was at least the size of my body, of stuff, and I can't believe it could be in there. But, see that is the classic regional enteritis disease. They've shot dye through people that have had it, and the lymph is totally congested and that shows in my eyes – the lymphatic rosary that's totally congested. You know, nothing hardly gets through, the colon is so layered with stuff. In autopsy, people with regional enteritis, their colon is just layers and layers of something. They don't even know what it is. They don't absorb foods, so they become thin and anemic and any disease can wipe them out and so I'm sure I've had a colon in this state for quite some time, plus tearing in the rectal area. It's a classic disease and it just showed in my eyes. But, back to the eye. It's so much different now."

Lavon: "How are you now?"

Gloria: "Well, there's not that heavy, heavy orange, showing on the iris of the eye, there's still some. Sometimes along the way I keep thinking, I've been on this a year, but I know people who have been on it for years and still have a long way to go, so I don't feel too badly. I have eaten a lot of the wrong combinations and a heavy protein diet because I always thought pork – lots of pork – and it's interesting, I've looked in the eyes of the people I've known from the south ever since, and I can't believe it. Their eyes are all orange. I know these people that raise pigs down in North Carolina, and I looked in their eyes and I couldn't believe it. Of course, I don't know if it were that exactly. But this one person's eyes I looked into, he's a good, good person. He's got all kinds of spots and orange. I notice eyes now."

Lavon: "You're thankful?"
Gloria: "Well, it's hard to say where I would be now. I know there was no way out. It was like a bottomless pit. This was the light I needed. I'm thankful, and if she listens to this tape she knows I'm thankful to her for what she's taught me."

Loretta Adams

This happened to my son who is seven years old, he had trouble all of his life since he was a baby with his bowels, and when he was about six he could only go to the bathroom about once a week and only with the suppository. I took him to the doctor, and he put him on mineral oil for two months. I had to give them 2 ounces every night of mineral oil, and it helped the condition. He got so he was going to the bathroom more, but I didn't notice until later, all but his vitamins and everything that he got from his food was going out with the mineral oil, and he got real bad strep infections that lasted for another couple of months after that. He would get them, we would get it almost cured, and then it was start back again. After he was off the mineral oil, he was all right for a month or two and then it started again, worse than before. He couldn't go to the bathroom so we took him back and the doctor took x-rays. In the lower bowel, in the sigmoid colon, there was a place that narrowed down to almost pencil thin and the doctor suggested that we bring him back, schedule him for a biopsy, and then to do surgery to remove that section of his colon. He said he didn't know what caused it, that it might be a part of his colon where the nerves weren't working.

We had him all scheduled for February for the operation, and about three weeks before the operation, I talked to a friend of mine who had been to some classes and she told me about the herbs, the herbal laxative, and the enemas and the things to do for it, and I thought well, I'll try anything because he had had several surgeries already in his life, and I didn't want him to have another one. So we gave him the enemas and the laxative. I gave him an herb laxative every day for a week and nothing happened. All of a sudden one

Sunday as we were getting him ready for Sunday school, he got sick. He had diarrhea, he started throwing up, and everything. I thought he just had the flu, but evidently this laxative finally started working on him, and I kept giving him a laxative and the enemas and then he had some bleeding, too. Red, fresh blood, so evidently the enemas had caused the bleeding, so I gave him goldenseal enema, and we worked on him like this for about three weeks. He was scheduled to go to the doctor for this biopsy, but they took x-rays first. I went over to the doctor's office. I had to go in first to talk over the x-rays with him before he went to the hospital, and he said, "I don't know what happened, but those areas are completely gone that he had on his colon." So he said, "I don't think there's any need to do the surgery or the biopsy, either one now."

Doctor Richard Storres

My name is Richard Storres. I'm 45 years old. Approximately 5 years ago I started to notice symptoms which I thought were of orthopedic origin, loss of function in my legs, which I later found out to be neurological and was finally diagnosed as multiple sclerosis. About three years ago I learned that I had diabetes and was started on Oranaz, an oral insulin, which later was changed to regular insulin shots, and approximately 2 months ago I was taking as much as 300 units of U-80 insulin – two shots in the morning, two shots in the evening to keep my diabetes under control and even then my tapes would often run +3 and +4.

In the meantime, my loss of function progressed to the point where I had to use a cane after about a year and a half and then a year after that I had to go to a walker. Just two months ago I was looking at the inevitability of ending up in a wheelchair permanently, and probably spending the rest of my life confined to a wheelchair.

Through four different people, I learned about LaDean Griffin and her mild food diet, and obtained the book entitled, *Is Any Sick Among You?*, Which I read several times and decided to launch myself on her program religiously.

After just 60 days, I have lost 32 pounds from 190 to 158, and I am able to get around much better than I did before for a long time; I am able to walk briefly for short periods at certain times without assistance whatsoever but the most important thing to me is I have been able to, for over a month, eliminate the need for insulin altogether. My tapes are completely negative and have been for over one month. As far as my expectations for the future, I expect and intend to follow this diet on a permanent basis and to eventually be able to walk normally once again and to regain my full health.

Lavon: "Isn't that a thrill to know that that's possible?"
Richard: "It certainly is. I never thought it was, but I've seen dramatic results in just a short period of time. I can imagine what would happen over a period of a year or two.

Lavon: "Oh, yes, I really believe in it. I think that I was led. I've prayed about it a lot. I really believe that I was led to the source and to become acquainted with LaDean Griffin."

Lavon: "Well, that's a thrill. Thanks very much, Richard."
Richard: "Thank you."

Shirley Story

I have a lot of little things to tell about, but the one main thing is kidney stones. I had suffered from kidney stones for a number of years. I've been hospitalized twice with them, so I knew what they were, and I kind of felt like the Lord sent this one on a Sunday just so I couldn't get hold of a doctor. But, I had gone down to church about three months ago, and in church I started getting this real severe pain, and I knew what it was, and by the time the church was over it was excruciating. I could hardly stand it. I went home and my husband frantically got on the telephone and started trying to call the doctor and couldn't reach him anywhere. In the meantime, I went in the bathroom and prayed about it for some kind of a feeling or an answer on what I should do. I don't know why. I hadn't even thought about LaDean's class that I had just taken last fall, but it came to me, anyway – LaDean's class – and that's all that came to me.

Lavon: "That was an answer to prayer."

Shirley: "Yes. Then I went to LaDean's book and started taking the juice of a lemon every time the pain hit, which was about 15 minutes."

Lavon: "Straight juice, or water with it?"

Shirley: "I mixed a little water with it about a fourth of a glass."

Lavon: "Almost straight?"

Shirley: "Yes. It was hard to down, but I made it. And I could see that the pain, it was getting less. I took this all day long until the pain was completely gone."

Lavon: "Maybe seven or eight times, you took it? Like every hour?"

Shirley: "Oh, I took it more than that. I took it every 15 minutes for a good two hours.

Lavon: "Is that right? Did it start to let up right away?"

Shirley: "No, not for a while, not for about two hours. And, in the meantime, my husband said, "You've got to go to the doctor. We're going to take you down. We've got to do something." And I said, "No, I want to try this because all he'll give his pain pills." So I stayed on this all day, and by the time night came I was not in too much pain. I could stand it."

Lavon: "There was a relief?"

Shirley: "Yes, and the next day it was gone. I didn't have any, so I went ahead and I took the formulas that she recommended for kidneys and then I stayed on just parsley – a parsley tea for about three days. I didn't eat anything, and I haven't had any more attacks."

Lavon: "That's wonderful, how many months has this been?"

Shirley: "It must be about three months."

Lavon: "Do you think you've passed the stone?"

Shirley: "I may have passed it or it was dissolved. That's what it does, it dissolves. She says in her book, it will dissolve it like water on rock salt."

Lavon: "Is that right?"

Shirley: "Yes. In fact, I take a little lemon juice once in a while when I think about it just to ward this off. It really works."

"My dad has Parkinson's disease. He went to an acupuncture doctor and had treatments and that didn't help. I've tried to talk to him and tried to get him on this mild food diet and raw juice diet and all the B vitamins, but he just can't see it so, finally he decided to go to the hospital and have some treatments. He was on ladulca, and it worked all right while he was in the hospital. We could see some difference, but after he got home in maybe two months time he started getting really deathly sick. He couldn't keep any food down. He was going downhill, losing weight, and the shaking was just worse. His whole body shook inside and everything, so finally I thought," Well, I've just got to face facts with him, you know, and say, Daddy, this isn't going to cure you, this isn't getting to the cause of it and you are wasting time." So this is what I did, and we finally have him on a real high B complex vitamin, and he's taking brewer's yeast, vitamin C, calcium and magnesium. He stopped taking the ladulca pills. He stopped taking them gradually. He doesn't take those now at all. His shaking has improved. He doesn't shake inside anymore. He says it feels so good not to be shaking inside. His thinking and everything has improved. He even got to a point where he couldn't drive, and his eyes were kind of starry. Now he's driving again. Well, that's a testimony for what food factors will do. Another thing, cayenne pepper. I've got a boy who is grown now, but when he was small, he had asthma so bad that we'd have to put them in the hospital – oxygen – to breathe, and this would come on in the winter or the fall when it was real wet. He seemed to be allergic or something to the dampness. So I had a friend that was apparently into the herbs, but I didn't realize it at the time so what she said went over my head, but she said," Shirley, please take cayenne pepper," so she fixed me some capsules, and I gave him those. I can't remember what the dosage was. But I started those in the late summer, and he didn't have another attack, and we gave him those all through his growing up years and he has never had another attack. Now he's in the Navy. He's out on a ship where it's really damp, and he doesn't have any problem.

134

Lavon: "Does he still take cayenne?"

Shirley: "He doesn't take any now. Well, that just really cured him of that. He had it so bad that his ribs hurt and he would shake and try to get air. Then after he took cayenne for maybe two or three weeks, he didn't have any more attacks, but I didn't let up. I kept giving them to him through the winter, and then as he grew up, each year in the fall I would start giving them to him."

Lavon: "It's really great. Do you have any more to tell me?"

Shirley: "No, I don't think so. Yes, I do. Yes, I do. With the vitamin C. About eight months ago I had a real severe earache and, of course, again I wasn't using my head, wasn't thinking. Well, I ran to the doctor, cause it was so bad I couldn't stand it. He made a culture and found out that it was an infection in my inner ear, and it was throwing my equilibrium out of balance, and I was working at a mill at the time. I could hardly stand the sounds of machines running, so I got on the medicine that he gave me. It seems to clear it up, and then again in maybe two weeks it came back. I was talking to my friend about it, and she said, "what about vitamin C?" So, I started taking vitamin C, 1000 mg every hour, and within two days it was cleared up. So, I keep lots of vitamin C in the house."

Lavon: "We should have a lot of C for storage. Is this the end of your testimony?"

Shirley: "Yes."

Lavon: "Well, thank you. That was great."

Arvilla Cox

My testimony has to do with colitis. I had problems; and I even thought it might also be ovary problems. I had pain in the lower stomach quite a while, I had this off and on. I didn't have any idea what it was, but at this time I was so sick that I decided, "I'm going to the doctor and find out what it is." I had already taken LaDean's class, but sometimes you decide you could treat it if you knew what treat, but you're not sure what you're treating, so I went to the doctor and they started running tests and decided, it might be colitis, but they weren't sure. They'd taken x-rays, so they put me on something – I don't even know what it was, it was ghastly. I came home and took it but nothing seemed to help. In these types of cases, you know, you can keep on hunting and then, back in for five days and see how you're doing and if that doesn't work, then we'll try something else so, this is exactly what I did. After 45 days I was still in bed. The fact is that I was so sore that for someone to sit on the bed that I was lying on, hurt. That jarring hurt me, and so I waited the five days and went back and they said, they had decided to try something else, so they gave me more medications and said, "Try this." So, I went home and this went on for three weeks. I was almost totally in bed or in the bathtub because I felt better in the bath, with heat or a hot water bottle. This is the way I was for three weeks and so I got up one morning and the doctors had just about decided it was colitis, so, I decided, I had taken LaDean's class, so what in the world am I going through all this for. I couldn't possibly do worse than the doctors. I decided this is the way it was going to go, so I got my slippery elm out. I had all these things, and I put the slippery elm in a capsule and I started taking it. I took it the first day, can't remember the amount it seems like it was about four capsules, every four hours.

Lavon: "Did you take okra?"

Arvilla: "I didn't even think about okra. I have slippery elm. I did real well, in fact, just that night I was feeling a little bit better, but I have to tell you, maybe this is the problem with all of us, we don't exactly stick to things. My daughter made a big pad of fudge the next day. This is one of the things, you know, diet, has so much to do with everything that we do. But I could not resist fudge, so the next day I had a few problems. But after the third day on slippery elm I was completely free of pain. I didn't have one bit more. I don't know what it does, but I'm a zealot when it comes to slippery elm. I'm not kidding. I'd shout from the top of the house tops because I still have problems once in a while. I can feel it coming on. I really wouldn't have believed that it was caused from stress as much as it is until I'll have things that bring on stress, and then I'll find it comes back as quick as I put myself under stress. When I do, I take slippery elm and by the next day I'm fine.

We have a lady in our area that was having a problem and she'd been to the doctors. Someone said, "Go talk to Arva. She is a slippery elm gal," so she came and talked to me. She asked me what I thought, and I said, "I can only tell you it works if it's colitis, because I know about that." I talked to her about two days later after she tried it she said she was feeling a lot better, and I've talked to her since and she doesn't have a problem. She has lost weight."

Lavon: "See how these testimonies help people learn?"

Arvilla: "I think this salve their talking about – this cancer removing salve is really great. You know, I can testify to the things that I've tried and I know. I think the whole thing is great, and I'm sure that it all works. But you know for a certainty when you've tried things and they work. I know my little boy has problems with boils. He loves to ride horseback and he has to ride bareback. He gets an infection, a boil and this salve they've got is great for drying. If I catch it when it's starting, within three days it's come to a head and it's over. In fact, you should have him give his testimony. If anything goes wrong, he says, "Just ask my mom. That works." I've got a few problems, but it was real funny when I was taking LaDean's class and I first started, she started teaching us these things. In these things I found out that cayenne pepper would work for ulcers, and I was having a lot of trouble with ulcers at the time. This is another stress type thing you know, and so this one night I was to go to class, and I hurt so bad, and I tried everything that I knew, like soda, and all the bad things that I tried and nothing worked and finally I called Bret and said," Bret, if you've got some capsules, bring them with you, or else I can't go to class." I said, "We'll give it a go. If I'm going to die, it will be down there with LaDean," because I was so afraid of it. You know if you've got an ulcer and you've talked to doctors you do not take spicy foods, and so I thought, "Okay, I'm going to put this to the supreme test because I'm taking two capsules of cayenne pepper," and I took it, and I went down and actually forgot to tell LaDean that I had taken it because I quit hurting, you know how you do when you're not hurting, you forget, and then it just quit. It just quit.

Lavon: "I hear a lot of good things about cayenne."

Arvilla: "I found that too. In fact, what are these kits were making an relief society? Safety kits? First aid kits, and we've been told – nurses are helping us get these little kits ready, and we've got all these neat things to put there in case of emergencies and in mine there is slippery elm and cayenne pepper and vitamin E. I have all these little extra things, these are the things we must store."

Lavon: "Well, Arvilla, I think your testimonies fantastic. It's going to help a lot of people. Thanks a lot."

Beryl Furner

At the time I was studying and taking classes from LaDean, I conversed with my sister about what I was learning. Because of my studies in iridology, I began to notice people's eyes and my sister's eyes were particularly interesting to me because she had one or two dark spots in each iris. I hesitated to talk to her about them, not knowing how she would accept it. After a few weeks I observed that one spot became larger and very dark.

My sister had complained of back problems and pain which she suspected to be gallbladder. Her doctor, after x-rays and checkup, told her he could offer no help or determination as to what the problem was or what to do about it so to let it go for a time. The spot grew larger. It was located in the right iris beginning in the ascending colon area and spread up into the shoulder area. The pain was in the upper right side of her back, under the shoulder. After hearing in class about a man with a similar problem and what he had done for it, I suggested to my sister, go on a mild food diet, take psyllium seed powder in water with laxative every night and also take a high enema each day for at least three days.

She continued with this treatment for two weeks. She noted the spot in her eye had faded. She told me she thought she had passed the bowel impaction. When I saw her after two weeks I detected no spot left in that area of her eye.

Gloria Wood

About my finger. I stuck my finger – my hand – in the sump pump, and it cut the fingers, the one real bad, and it was sewer water. It was open, so it got an infection in it. We cleaned it out and used this cancer formula, and it has done wonders. It drew all the infection out. We just kept putting it on it. It left a scar, but it closed it right off and helped it beautifully. In fact, as my husband says, "That would make a believer out of anybody." Just a few days and it was great, well about a week, it was a deep cut, and it really did wonders. I have two boys that have ulcers and I have ulcers. We use slippery elm and okra, the minute their stomachs even think they're going to hurt. Another one is goldenseal and myrrh. That does wonders for trench mouth or cold sores or canker sores. My son had trench mouth so bad, he had it clear down the back of his throat and all out on his neck. He couldn't even eat, he had to suck through a straw, it was so bad. He rinsed his mouth with goldenseal and myrrh and it just did wonders.

Veva Whitear

Lynn: "Veva, we'd like to hear your testimony. We hear that you've had a little girl and she's been much improved since you've had her on mild foods and licorice root."

Veva: "Our little girl has hypoglycemia. When I first suspected she had it, she would wake up in the morning when she was just a baby. Then I would give her a bottle and her little hands would shake so bad that she could hardly hold it. She needed food. Her blood sugar level was low. When she got about three years old, in the morning when she woke up if we didn't have food immediately the first thing she would do would be shake. The next thing she would do is say, "My stomach hurts." The next thing she would do – I knew I had about 10 seconds and she would feel like she was going to vomit and then she would pass out.

When we went to the doctors, they kind of pooh-poohed this hypoglycemia and they wondered why I thought this was the problem, and I told him because it ran in the family. Her father, some 20 years ago, had a problem and he had done the same thing in the morning when he'd been without food all night and the blood sugar level was low. He'd go out and milk and do chores before he had any breakfast and if I didn't have some food for him in a hurry all at once he become terribly ill and he would pass out. His family thought he either had a tumor on his pancreas or it was hypoglycemia. It turned out to be hypoglycemia. But when I took my little girl to the doctor he said, "Well, what makes you think she has this problem?" I said,

"Because she reacts just like her father reacted some years ago; he doesn't have the problem now, apparently he is balanced now. His sister has the problem also." They pooh-poohed it. They said, "Little children don't have this so much and it's kind of a fad thing these days."

One day in a dentist's office she got scared because she's afraid of the sight of blood. They had to pull a root of a tooth out that she had broken off. She became so upset she passed out. So, she doesn't have normal balance and cannot take stress. I took her immediately to the doctor, a pediatrician – and he said," Oh, I don't think we need to worry about that. When I was a kid I used to pass out when I got scared, too."

At Christmas time she had had a bunch of sweets at a party at school – this was when she was in kindergarten. When she came home she was running around the table with her little friend who was visiting and she fell and hit the corner of the stereo right on her knee and it hurt her severely and she went into convulsions. I decided then, "Oh, boy, we've got real problems." Passing out and convulsions and I didn't know what this convulsions bit was. I called the doctor and he sent me to a neurologist. When I went to him they put her in the hospital and ran tests, costing us a lot of money, and they couldn't come up with anything that was wrong with her. I kept telling him I knew she had hypoglycemia, and he said, "This convulsions thing – well, we don't know what that is. I have about 10 children a month and they hit themselves and they go into a convulsion. It doesn't happen to older people, it happens to children." But he was concerned about this other – passing out and so forth. When he got through with the test he said, "Well, it didn't show anything." He was worried about epilepsy, it didn't really show this by the tests he took, but he put her on Dilantin. I was just so sure that he hadn't come up with what was wrong and I knew what was wrong. I went down to the health store and started talking to them. I got a Adelle Davis' book and I started reading in there and it gave all of her symptoms, even to the part of convulsions when they have this problem, and so I threw away the Dilantin and started her on some vitamins at that time. I hadn't met LaDean then. I found our neighborhood had classes that LaDean taught.

Lynn: "Did the vitamins help a lot, though?"

Veva: "Yes, they did help a lot. It wasn't the whole answer yet. She was still shaky every once in a while, and I had to be very careful with her, and when there were stress, times when she was really frightened, I had to be careful. After I took the class from LaDean and found out about the licorice root, I just started her with licorice root. I wasn't convinced at this particular time, but I started her anyway."

Lynn: "Is she taking any other herbs?"

Veva: "No, she's taking vitamins. She takes potassium, magnesium, vitamin B6, B complex, etc."

Lynn: "Is she taking a lot of C?"

Veva: "No, I haven't given her C. I was giving her some kelp. I thought this would hurt, but, you know, she got high strung and she got really nervous. I thought, "Something I'm doing is wrong." I kept thinking about kelp having to do with the thyroid, and I thought, "I wonder if she's getting too much and making her nervous." It is natural thyroid, and I took the kelp away from her and she is fine."

She did so well for a while, we kind of decided, well, maybe she's outgrowing this, so after a while, we ran out of vitamins and I didn't get them. She did really well for about six months and we had no more problem. We thought maybe she was over this problem. Last March she and an older sister decided they wanted to get me and my husband an anniversary present, and they didn't have the money, being little children, but they wanted to give us something nice. They decided they would go without their lunch at school to save their lunch money for the gift. Well, the first part of April she had been going without meals which she shouldn't do with low blood sugar. One morning she got up, she hadn't had a problem now for three years. She was practicing piano and all at once she jumped up and started running to the kitchen. She felt a pain in her stomach she knew, she just had a few minutes to get something in her stomach or she would pass out. As soon as she got to the end of the couch she fell on the floor. She tried to get up, but she couldn't. All at once it donned on me, "Here we are." I ran to the kitchen to get something fast, but it was too late. She said, "I'm going to throw up." Then she passed out and went into a convulsion. This was after she had been going without meals for nearly a month."

Lynn: "She learned a lesson there, didn't she?"
Veva: "Really, and so did we. We got her back on herbs. She is really on a program now, and doing fine."

Jan Perry

We've been on mild food about seven months now. We really feel like it's helped us. I for myself, feel like this method has saved my life. I was told I had leukemia and I feel now that it is on the mend.

Lynn: "Have you been on it strictly, the mild foods?"
Jan: "Pretty strict. We've eaten a few things now and then, as most people probably do, pretty strict on mild foods. I've used psyllium, the CS formula, liquid dulse, licorice and Lobelia."

Lynn: "Have you noticed a big change in your eyes?"
Jan: "It's really hard for me to compare my eyes with the slide, I'm anxious to have our eye slides taken again and compare. I feel like there is a change in my eyes. I feel so much better than I did before I started."

Lynn: "Did you have any specific problems, other than leukemia?"
Jan: "I've had female problems and when I look at my eyes, I wonder what I don't have."

Lynn: "How's your family taking to this?"
Jan: "My family really has accepted this well."

Lynn: "Have they done pretty well, too?"
Jan: "Yes. One problem we have is they're tired quite a bit, but I guess that's due to eliminating. At least, I feel like they are. I'm really glad that my whole family has accepted this.

Last summer I went to the doctor and my blood was real low, and for a period of about three months I kept going back. He'd check it every week, every two or three weeks, and he kept giving me iron shots and iron pills and all kinds of things, and he was very alarmed that my blood didn't come back up. At this time I was told that I had a leukemia condition, and that's when I started on the mild food, and I have felt so much better that I really have a testimony that it's right."

Elaine Thompson

I have a boy who is retarded and he's also epileptic. When he was two days old, he started having seizures. I didn't get him out of the hospital until he was two weeks old, and he was put on phenobarbital. We had them on that for a while and phased him off and he was fine. He didn't have another seizure until he was 11 years old, and then he started having them again. I took him to the Oregon Medical Center. I've had him to several neurologists. I've had him to one in Ogden. I've had him to the University of Utah Medical Center, and no matter what they gave him, it didn't control it. He was so drugged at one time that he couldn't walk a straight line down the hall at school. It just made me sick to watch him because he was – well, you know, it's bad enough when he's retarded, but having this on top of it. It really bothered me – so, when I heard about this class of LaDean's, I thought, "Well, gee, that might be some way to help him."

Lavon: "Do I understand you now that you've had him on drugs up to this point?"
Elaine: "Up to this point, yes, where I came to LaDean's class. In fact he was taking Dilantin and then he was taking something stronger than that, and I can't remember what it was. He was also taking something stronger than the phenobarbital. It was about the strongest things they could give him. He was taking about two or three of them.

Lavon: "Did he act drugged up when he took those?"
Elaine "Oh, yes, he was really, really drugged up. Besides that, they have a lot of trouble with their gums with the Dilantin, unless they keep their mouths real clean. I've always had trouble getting him to brush his teeth. But anyway, I took the class and so I decided I

would take him off the drugs, the Dilantin and the other drug. I replaced it, four to one – four nervine herb tablets and one of the other kind and then I gave him B complex and calcium – four of each to one of the white pills that he had. As I upped the nervine and B complex, I lowered the other, so I didn't do it all at once. It wasn't just a straight cut off. I combined them at first and then I gradually took him off all of the drugs. He's been off them for more than a year and a half.

Lavon: "He isn't a bit worse?"

Elaine: "No, he's really better. When I first got him off of it, when he'd have a spell, he'd really be sick and I decided maybe it was withdrawal from the other drug, because he'd be sick for maybe twelve hours after. He was sick to his stomach and would throw up and now he's gotten to the point, though he still has some seizures, he has them mostly at night and he doesn't get sick like he used to. He still has to sleep them off, but he's so much more alert and he's so much more easy to work with because he isn't drugged up. He just looks like it. You could see the look on his face. Well, that's the way my boy was."

Lavon: "Then you really are thankful for this way of life, aren't you?"

Elaine: "Oh, yes, I wouldn't go back to the other for anything. I think if I can get him on the right diet. He's 18 now and he doesn't like to be on a mild food diet. I think if I could get him on that kind of food that it would lessen it a lot.

I also have one other thing to tell you. I have a daughter that gets earaches quite often. About a year ago, she had a real bad ear infection. In fact, she couldn't stand up. It seemed like an inner ear infection so I just kept her on high vitamin C, and I rubbed her glands. She also had swollen glands and I rubbed them with an iodine salve and kept cold packs on her ears, and she was over it in about two or three days, which was probably a shorter time than it would have been on antibiotics to get over it because an inner ear infection can go on for a week or two.

144

Vitamin C is a fantastic thing this was 1000 units every hour and whenever the kids are sick, that's what I say, "Okay, 1000 units every hour." Vitamin C and juice. I forgot to say I've got Gary on vitamin C 3000 mg. a day, he takes B complex and B$_6$, magnesium and just about everything. Well, just about anything I hear of that's helped an epileptic person I start giving it to him and I think they all kind of help him. He used to be quite sickly, but now he's hardly ever sick."

Hawley Haws

I'm just beginning to learn a little bit about herbs but what I have learned so far I'm really excited about, because I'm able to help myself and my children and my husband without running to the doctor the first little thing that comes along. First of all, when my last little baby was just tiny, I brought her home from the hospital, she had a rash on her bottom right from the start and I put paper diapers on her, so it wasn't a matter of diaper rash. It was some other type of rash she picked up at the hospital, and I tried everything. All the normal creams that were on the market.

Finally, I went back to the doctor because it was just a blistering low rash and very sore and he gave me a prescription which was a 7$ or 9$ tube with about a quarter of an ounce of cream and that would begin to almost burn the skin till it was just kind of cauterizing it, but then the rash would come back immediately after. So that wasn't doing a thing. And then I read in one of the books that I have – I don't remember what it was – that goldenseal was a real good thing for skin rash and other skin conditions. I used it just on the clean bottom all by itself, instead of baby powder and overnight the little bottom began to dry up and the blisters cleared up within the next couple days. Now whenever I have a problem of the rash coming back at all I just put a little of the goldenseal on it and then leave the little bottom open to the dry air during the day as much as possible and it really does the trick it heals it so quickly, I was amazed.

We've also used goldenseal on canker sores and other skin lesions and then I discovered, thanks to my aunt LaDean's book, that catnip tea is real good for colic, and I've used it with the last couple of babies and had almost no problem with colic. The catnip tea tends to be just a little bit bitter, so I put a little bit of honey with it and a little bit of alfalfa mint tea or another mild tea with it. I've also used comfrey tea as a cleansing tea for my smaller children to help get rid of colds or flu quickly because the other teas tend to be a little bit strong for their little systems.

Now the real thing that was a testimony to me about herbs and vitamins and cleansing diet, was when I got hepatitis, a rare type called Primary Cholangiolitic hepatitis. My whole skin would itch and I turned yellow, of course, but the main problem with hepatitis is that it can cause permanent damage to the liver and kidneys if it's not taken care of properly, and I knew I had to have complete bed rest. Since I had four small children, my mother came and took care of the two smaller children while I just stayed completely in bed. Then my sister took the two older children with her. I had heard that with this disease you must have complete hospital rest for six weeks to two months. I expected that I would have a serious problem getting myself back on my feet. In fact with this kind of hepatitis, I was told that there would be approximately 2 years to recuperate, where I would have my complete strength back, and I knew that I couldn't afford that with all my family's needs.

With the help of my mother and aunt LaDean's book which we consulted because she knew more about herbs and about nutrition for ailments than my mother did, I began an herb program. My mother knew enough to put me immediately on a complete fast first and then gradually I would have vitamin C at high potency and with help from my aunt LaDean's book, I took lemon juice and water with no sweetening in it, about every hour during the day, along with the high potency vitamin C about every hour, I had about 1000 to 2000 mg every hour. I had vitamin A and vitamin E and I took vitamin B complex because I was taking goldenseal and they need to work together. I also was taking the CS formula because they are excellent cleansing herbs, and this is what I needed to do, get that all out of my system before it could do any damage to my organs. I also took another formula, I don't remember the name of it, especially for cleansing the liver and kidney which were the two that were affected the most by the hepatitis.

It was really amazing. I knew that I would be over the hepatitis enough to get out of bed soon. The yellow was completely gone and out of the whites in my eyes as well. Within about 2 1/2 weeks that was completely gone, and here I had expected it would go on for six weeks to two months, and then within another year I was completely back with my energy back and my strength and I gradually brought fruits and vegetables into my diet and now have my full strength. I am expecting our fifth child and I feel better with this pregnancy than I remember ever feeling before. I've had no morning sickness, and I really think that the cleansing has helped this pregnancy to be better and to be easier. I'm really happy that I have aunt LaDean, and that her book could help me and that I had the help of my sweet mother and sister.

Bessie Upwall

For the last 4 1/2 to 5 years, I have had a real bad colitis problem. In June 1974, I was advised by two doctors to quit my job because of pressures. I wasn't getting enough rest and was working too hard. They advised me that I would never be any better if I didn't give up my job. I quit my job for a year and a half and it was then I met Lavon Thomas. She introduced me to herbal living. I read LaDean's book about herbs and decided that that was the way I wanted to go.

I started taking herbs four or five months ago. I took saffron, slippery elm, black walnut, psyllium, the CS formula, capsicum and I've also been taking a combination of hops, Valerian root and skullcap. I think that has helped me more than any, if I were to say one herb combination was the one that really helped me the most. It has helped my colon to remain calm along with everything else. Then I went on a strict diet, left meat alone, ate vegetables, fruits and so on. I not only got my colon better but I lost 13 pounds. I'm still trying to eat right. If I cheat and eat some things I'm not supposed to then I suffer a little bit but nothing like before.

I'm now holding down a job again, which the doctors said I probably never would be able to, having lots of energy, being able to do the things I need to do and feeling better than I felt in five years.

Lavon: "Isn't that great. You attribute it all to the herbs?"

Bessie: "You bet I do because I haven't felt this good in that long and I know that nothing else has helped me before.

Lavon: "Do you feel that in another month or two your colon will probably be well?"

Bessie: "Yes and I might add too, that I was going every three or four months to Wyoming to a doctor and he was doing adhesion work on me. When I was there in December, I had only been on the herbs two or three months and he said that it was better than it had been in years. I hope to be able to lengthen out my visits now and possibly not have to go back again."

Lavon: "So you're a real herb fan?"

Bessie: "You bet and I thoroughly believe in capsicum because boy that really is a healer and sure gives you a lot of energy. I take it faithfully."

Lavon: "Do you?"

Bessie: "You bet. Oh, I might add another thing about black cohosh; also in 1974 – in June – I had a breast that was weeping and the doctor had to cut me way back on my estrogen and said I may have to go off of it completely. I wasn't able to go off of it completely because of other symptoms I had then. When I started on black cohosh, I was able to cut my estrogen way back and take the black cohosh and now my breast is completely cleared up."

Lavon: "Is that right, and how long did you have that?"

Bessie: "I had it for two years."

Lavon: "So you think black cohosh did it?"

Bessie: "Oh I know it did because its helped to balance my estrogen and let me cut way back on the other estrogen product that I was taking and I've felt great. I haven't had a lot of hot flashes or depression or anything like I had before."

Lavon" And you've really been through a lot of things too."

Bessie: "I sure have."

148

Lavon: "A lot of stress?"

Bessie: "Yes, a lot of stress and strain, I've been going through a divorce."

Lavon:" Your testimony is going to mean a lot to people that read this book."

Bessie: "I hope so because I know that without herbs, I would be where I was several months ago, only worse, because of all the stress I've been under. I would really have been down the tube if it hadn't been for those herbs."

Lavon: "One thing that I can appreciate about you Bessie is that you take them regularly and the way you should and drink plenty of water. If people would just stick with the program, they would see results."

Bessie: "That's true. I found that if I stay with it really faithfully, I just feel great and I get along good. Like I said, if I cheat on it, I eat sweets or if I eat meat very much – once in a while if I eat a little chicken or something like that it doesn't bother me, but I try not to do that."

Lavon: "Eat a beefsteak or anything?"

Bessie: "I haven't had a stake in months and months. If I eat anything that has very much meat in it, I really suffer, that or heavy sweets. So I know that those two things I really have to leave alone or eat very, very sparingly. If I just stick to fruits and vegetables, I just get along great."

Lavon:" Okay, thanks a lot Bessie."

Linda Beal

When I was young I didn't pay much attention to the Word of Wisdom except for no smoking, no drinking. Always when I read the Doctrine and Covenants section 89, I felt that I was doing right, meat could be eaten any time, herbs and that advice were for people in Moses' time.

As I went through my 24 years of life, ate all things that I wanted, when I wanted, I had all childhood diseases. I was always sick, with sore throats, ear aches, constipation. I had terrible cramping when my periods would start then less period and more cramping, more often – three times a month. I used a bottle syringe for a full year because I didn't have any other way of relief of constipation.

My cousin told me about mild food diet and how it could heal your body. I believed everything she told me that day. I started immediately, left my second glass of cocoa and four pieces of toast and lunch of Dr Pepper and candy bars alone. I thought," Really I'll eat better now than I ever have." I had had a terrible pain in my left side and went to the doctor. I had x-rays, wasting a lot of time and money and he said, "Can't see anything wrong with you." Something had to be wrong, you don't have three periods a month and constipation that bad for no reason, no wonder I felt sick.

I ate mild foods and herbs, psyllium, lower bowel herbs, CS, female corrective herbs, nervine herbs. Miraculous things began to happen immediately. Bowels were already working better. I don't use anything like a bottle syringe anymore. I have good periods and they are regular. I felt like I was alive with lots of energy. I could read and not fall asleep.

I lived for four months on mild foods. It took me four months of living like this, then my body went through a healing crisis. You really feel sick with it. It lasted only one day and I felt like a million the next day. I try and live on a mild food diet and take herbs occasionally. I feel really good now. I know it's the truth.

Rich Wheeler

By the time I was 24 years old in 1962, refined carbohydrates, principally sugar, had severely damaged my health. I had developed hypoglycemia. Unfortunately, it was a full 13 years, before the correct diagnosis was finally made. Those 13 years were filled with crushing medical bills, dozens of "specialists" and myriads of negative test results.

Prior to that time I was a regular guy: happy, fun loving, always quick to laugh. I seldom worried about anything. You can imagine how disconcerting it was for me to find myself constantly worrisome, and fearful. Equally disquieting where the ever present headaches, mental confusion, abdominal cramps and inner trembling. I was sure the local doctor could help me find the problem. Many x-rays and several dollars later, the physician indicated that the promised ulcer was not there. Nervous stomach was pronounced the culprit. However, the symptoms didn't leave as readily as my money had. The answer was obvious, try the specialists in the big city.

I went the full route. There were chiropractic adjustments, eyeglass fittings, dental spacing plates and tests and tests and tests at the clinic. The medics pronounced me clean, gave me a bottle of tranquilizers and wished me well. Think of it; my very first bottle of tranquilizers!

The summer of '63 found me newly married and living in Tucson, Arizona. The tranquilizers were ineffective and I kept driving my tired body as best I could wondering, "Why me"? In August '64 an expert diagnostician, of which there were plenty in Tucson, prescribed Bellergral space tabs to alleviate my symptoms. It seemed to help with success was short-lived.

Acute pancreatitis landed me in the hospital in September. I was elated to have a real disease. It was good to know at last the cause of those terrible pains in the abdomen. Once the crisis was over I was dismissed without even so much as a word of counsel. The stage for the next crisis was thus set.

Early in 1965, two different cardiologists heard suspicious noises in my neck. An arteriogram was ordered and three days later the customary negative results were given to me. After contracting hay fever in '66 the summer of '67 introduced me to acute prostate infection which was to plague me for years. The Bellergral tranquilizer carried me nicely through the spring of '69 but I hated my dependence on it. Instinctively, I had cut down gradually and eventually decided to stop altogether.

During the summer long working hours, extreme mental stress and poor eating habits reduced my weight drastically. In October it happened! Uncontrollable body tremors and anxieties that could only be described as pure horror. Once again I reached out for the arm of flesh for help. Luckily for me my physician was acquainted with the "best" psychiatrist in Salt Lake City.

Along with psychotherapy, the doctor tried me on several drugs to take care of the anxiety-depression reaction I had experienced. In spite of the fact that no insomnia was present a powerful sleep inducing drug called Parest was administered. I slipped rapidly into depression. For over a month I was apathetic, lethargic and constantly obsessed by suicidal thoughts. Sinequan, a new drug, was given because it had" uppers" and "downers" both. But the mainstay was to be the wonder drug, Valium, relatively new but unquestionably safe. Valium and I were to see many years come and go together.

In 1970 I began losing great amount of hair. At the same time I came to enjoy the toxic effect of the Parest even though the doctor had cautioned me about it. My body weight moved up to a peak of 200 pounds then slowly descend into my normal of 175. By the summer of '72 I was in terrible physical condition weighing only 168 pounds (I am 6'6"). To correct this I began to work out with weights and take a high-protein anti-stress formula ala Adele Davis. The results were impressive, I gained 20 pounds of good solid muscle and rapidly increased my muscular strength. The only problem was the growing intensity of those same abdominal cramps and raw eczema on the hands and feet. Before I could take evasive action, the pancreas inflamed again and I was hospitalized. I was sick with worry. After dismissal from the hospital I found that concentrated use of the B complex vitamin cleared up the hands and feet in about two weeks.

There was no improvement in my general health but with the help of Valium, I was at least able to hold onto my job as a landscape architect. I was never far from the "wonder drug" and would never leave the house without padding my pocket to see that my friend was there. I was just plain hooked! I wanted off but the doctor discouraged me and also I lacked the personal courage and faith to do it.

Eventually, however, I was forced to resign my government post after 12 years of service. The quality of my work was high but the quantity was too low, the boss said. The truth was that I just didn't care about my work anymore.

In June '74 the prostate flared up again. We treated it with sulfa drugs. Then, to "take care" of my hay fever, I took a Kenalog shot. I felt fairly good through the summer. Pancreatitis struck again early in September and down I went once more. A week later the prostatitis manifest itself again. Tests indicated that I was anemic because of a shortage of hemoglobin. I experienced general apathy, fatigue and depression throughout that fall. The prostate infection submerged and then resurfaced in April. Antibiotic drugs were now totally ineffective and my strength waned. I realized by mid-June, '75 that I was seriously ill.

As the impending crisis loomed before me I knelt in prayer before my Heavenly Father to seek His counsel. Much to my amazement and chagrin, the Lord specifically instructed me to "get off medication". I was shocked! Didn't He realize how sick my body was? Why did He wish an additional problem on me at a time like this? I knew that I was addicted to Valium and that getting off would mean additional stress to my failing body. To say that I was frightened would be a gross understatement of fact. After wrestling with my faith for a couple of days and "delaying" my usual dosage just long enough to experience discomfort, I felt my cause was hopeless. The Father, always patient, spoke to me again through one of His servants. I was told that as I gained control of my own body, the desires of my heart would be granted. I knew then that He stood ready to help me accomplish that which He had commanded. I promised Him that I would stop taking the drug.

Hell yawned wide and I was swallowed up. Hallucinations, phobias, muscle twitching, pain and no sleep where the order of the day as my body cried out for its accustomed poison. Fortunately I was led by the Spirit to a doctor who ministered to his patients with natural extracts, vitamins, minerals, herbs and mild foods. He was very helpful in the struggle to preserve my life. In addition to drug withdrawal and the underlying infection throughout my body, I had developed hemorrhoids, a protein deficiency, several mineral deficiencies, hypothyroidism, sluggish adrenal glands, digestive insufficiency, anemia, back pains, numerous allergies and, of course, I still had the ever present low blood sugar. Together with my faithful wife I prayed day and night for deliverance.

Even as hell yawned, the windows of heaven opened above us. Blessings poured down upon our heads beyond our ability to contain them. For two weeks we were taught by the Lord. Many of the spiritual gifts mentioned in the Scriptures became ours. Where doubt had existed faith now stood. We knew that He lived. Being driven to our knees, as it were, the Father took our outstretched hand and led us daily.

It took another four weeks for the drug to be cleansed from my body to the point where I was reasonably comfortable some of the time. I experienced crushing headaches throughout the balance of the summer of '75 and the prostate problem gave me little relief. I grew impatient with the Lord and pled for Him to heal me immediately. I knew He had the power to do so; I just couldn't understand why He didn't.

The mild food diet was tough to stay on. Old habits crept back and, while I never touched refined sugar, I did occasionally take some meat and practically lived on whole wheat bread at times. However, a bounteous fruit crop supplied me with lots of fresh produce in season. I enjoyed, in turn, the cherries, apricots, pears, peaches, prunes and apples, consuming large amounts. As fall neared I was strong enough to engage in a few physical activities. Then the adrenals sagged even lower and back to bed I went. I found that the adrenals were particularly weak in the late afternoon, usually creating a crisis. Then about 1:00 to 3:00 AM, I would awaken as they hit their low point of hormone production. At such times, there was difficulties in breathing and my chest muscles seemed partially paralyzed. Life wasn't rewarding at all. All this was attended by much mental confusion, depression and I often found myself crying at the least provocation. I wondered if I would ever really get well; I guess my faith was near an all-time low. I had little or no patience with my children and wasn't particularly kind to my wife.

Since I hadn't worked in a regular job in 2 years, our financial situation was precarious at best. Miraculously, the Lord open ways for us to be provided for and we never have been deprived. Our housing was less than adequate so as winter approached we began to look for a new home where it would be possible to juice vegetables, bake bread, sit in the sun and do other things necessary to getting well.

In December we moved to southern Utah. After getting settled in and after having recovered from the extreme stress of moving, I became really serious about my mild food diet. Right along I had been faithful in taking my adrenal cortial extract, licorice root, goldenseal, and various cleansing and rejuvenating herbs as well as large amounts of vitamin C, B complex, etc. At Christmas time I started pushing lettuce, celery and carrots juice. I was very kind to my pancreas and ate mostly fresh fruits, vegetables and raw nuts. After about 2 to 3 weeks on this regimen I began to notice a strange thing happen. My mental powers were returning! My intellectual appetite became enormous and I began to read more and more with increasing retention of what I read. Even more exciting, however, I sensed my spirituality growing. I now realize, in retrospect, that this Spirit of the Lord certainly cannot operate to any great degree in an unclean tabernacle. Even though my body was getting stronger, I recognized that improvement in my physical health would be a pace or two behind the mental and spiritual. That was fine for me for now, I realized that I would eventually be completely healed and enjoy a degree of health hitherto unknown to me. For certainly, God cannot lie.

I know that all of my problems as outlined above came upon me because I violated the Laws of God. First, I ravaged my body for several years with excessive refined carbohydrates like sugar and white flour. Next I didn't meet the results of that mistake with faith but literally "worried myself sicker". Thirdly, and this also pertains to a lack of faith, I placed myself in the hands of uninspired doctors who almost destroyed my bodily organs with drugs through ignorance. I never plan to repeat these costly errors but, at the same time, I am joyous over the spiritual experience I gained.

Looking back at those dark days, I realize that the Lord spared my life by directing me to get off of drugs. I am grateful He loved me that much. I am thankful that He had enough confidence in my wife and to guide us to many truths. I have great joy when I reflect upon the experiences we had together, many of which are too sacred to relate here in. One of these experiences I came to know and know now that He lives! He lives! I know that He lives and that Jesus is His Christ, that these revelations are open and available to all who seek Him. I know that if we develop the faith and the courage to try His ways that we can all have these gifts.

The Lord has not placed us here on the earth to wander in ignorance. His Law of Health is available to us through the Scriptures, through inspiration and through His chosen servants. If we will but heed that which we have been given and not violate the laws of God, we will have health in the navel and marrow in the bone. This I know. This I can never deny.

I am grateful for this testimony that I have, and pray that I might never do anything that would violate it and that I might endure to the end with my family and be exalted in the Celestial Kingdom of God. This I say humbly bearing witness to all that I have said, in the name of Jesus Christ, Amen.

Sandy Eggerson

I am giving this testimonial to show how people can improve their health without having to go through all the operations and drugs. I've been ill for most of my life and not able to find out what was wrong; going from doctor to doctor. I have had several accidents and never any extreme illnesses, just not well.

I went to LaDean's classes before her book was even printed or published, the first series, that she ever gave. It was on herbs and then I started on herbs and juices and various things. I started cleansing at different periods of time. Then I went to the iridology classes she discussed how you can find different things in the eye. I decided that I would try some of the things that were useful for the different places that I saw in my own eye. One of the main things was parasites and there was indication of possible cancer. The first thing I did was use the CS formula. I used oil of wintergreen, taking four drops each day for 10 days and abstaining for 20 days and then taking it again for 10 days. During this time I ate a fairly normal diet of vegetables and fruits and some bread, some cereals. During this time I passed at least three different growths, cancerous type growths that we can tell for sure. Then numerous, I couldn't say how many, probably at least 100 roundworms and five or six tapeworms.

Lavon: "Sandy, what we want to stress now is that you left meat alone didn't you?"
Sandy: "Yes."

Lavon: "And how about sugars and starches?"
Sandy: "Oh we've been off sugar for several years and no meat."

Lavon: "Did you go on the cleansing herbs?"
Sandy: "Yes and I used cayenne, the CAC formula, Lobelia and black walnut. The herbal pumpkin didn't do as well for me. I just was too full of toxins and poisons and so I had to use garlic enema to help clean my body to help get the poisons out so that I wouldn't cleanse too fast. I don't know how many masses of worms etc. There was one time that I had a blockage because a mass had moved in the colon but we were able to get that out too. I wasn't even able to walk from the house to the garden. I wasn't able to do housework or even my dishes, it was just awful."

Lavon: "Strings of mucus came forth?"
Sandy: "Oh yes but the worms were fairly whole. I had the ability someway to cast them off and the growths too, the cancerous growths, came out most of them in one mass. Some of them had to break and rupture before I could pass them because they were too large. Your body can take care of just about everything if you can work with it and do the right things for it. I am very convinced that you do not have to go through all the drugs and operations unless you have been so seriously injured in a car accident, like a leg was amputated or something like this where the body cannot handle it where there is just too much destruction done. You can't expect that kind of a miracle but if the body is able to function, and my liver

wasn't functioning. My kidneys were doing fairly well, the pancreas still is not functioning properly. I had severe hypoglycemia."

Lavon: "You used the licorice?"
Sandy: "Yes, I used licorice root and don't even need it anymore. I have gotten to the point where my body is working on its own and the licorice root just isn't needed now."

Lavon: "You couldn't go strictly fruit either, you would cleanse too fast."
Sandy:" No, I couldn't because I nearly died. I was drowning in my own waste."

Lavon: "So the mild foods is better to help to slow that down so you won't cleanse too fast?"
Sandy: "Yes. We don't use any type of dairy products now and we don't use meat and no sugars or starches, things like this. Everyone is a lot better."

I'm very thankful for the whole thing, for LaDean and for her books and all that she has researched.

> *"A profound study of the law of cause and effect is the foundation of wisdom.*
> *J. Melvin Gibby*

CHAPTER 4

IT WORKS

Know ye not that your body is the temple of the Holy Ghost which is in you, which you have of God, and ye are not your own?

1 Corinthians.6:19

If a man defile the temple of God, him shall God destroy, for the temple of God is holy, which temple ye are.

1 Corinthians3:17

Through small beginnings, such as giving proof of the use of mild food and herbs by what takes place in the eyes, could bring our society to a point where organic food would be available everywhere, followed by herbs and natural vitamins. The knowledge of correct food combinations and sound principles regarding diet would then be taught in the schools. It could also be that sickness will be looked upon with contempt rather than with sympathy as it was in ancient Israel when sickness was considered a sin. We may then be asked, when we are sick, "What have you been eating?"

Following a lecture I gave in Los Angeles recently a man came up to me after the class and said, "I've heard you say this so many times in your classes I thought you would like to have this." He handed me a badge with two words on it, "It Works." After giving it some thought, I realized that I was saying, "It Works", repeatedly simply because it **does** work. My own personal experience in addition to the experiences of hundreds of people over many years I have studied the human body and natural methods have not always witnessed me **how** it works; but with great conviction I have witnessed that it **does** work. Recently, by way of fumbling around for an explanation of how it works, I have heard people say – and even some have written – that it works merely on the principle of faith or belief in the herbs and mild food, or faith in whoever is teaching these principles. We have not looked long enough nor intelligently enough at how the body feeds and eliminates if we are willing to brush aside so great a truth with an "It's all in your mind" attitude. When the same herbs have worked for the same ailments for the many generations since written records have existed, and because they work equally as well on babies as they do on mature people, it logically follows that a change must occur, a final result that is caused by the correct answer to a given health problem.

Mathematically, sociologically and scientifically there are laws which dictated given effect for a given cause. Why would the universe exist in such beautiful order if the human body were just a hodgepodge of chance? Some who live on the premise that the mind can do anything by just thinking positively, still die; and it would be with difficulty that they grow back a leg that had been cut off, no matter how much they thought about it. Problem is that everyone becomes "too soon old and too late smart." By the time a family is raised, the knowledge of how to raise children is grasped. Relatively late in life one begins to bring correct values into better focus. However, the problem of computed habit patterns in the brain, which started out like a fine thread, have been woven into a huge rope too difficult to break. Sometimes the only thing that makes it possible to sever this tie to bad habit is fear or pain, so that when the time seems ripe and the body is racked with pain as well as threatened with death, the struggle to loosen the body from the clutches of broken law begins. This is exactly what it amounts to – broken law. Perhaps not all the laws were broken that have brought the body to such a place of degradation. Was it a wayward child? Was it a miserable husband or wife? Was it financial circumstances? Was it war or famine? Was it a hateful boss or grandparents? The Lord said he would visit the sins of the parents on the children even unto the fourth generation. Was it ancestors who have caused suffering? Tests with rats have shown that an incorrect diet can affect posterity of the animal for many as four generations. In all fairness to those who come after us, isn't it time we did something to help ourselves as well as our children by learning and living the law upon which good health is predicated?

The discovery of laws is the beginning of wisdom. To live by them brings perfection – a perfect knowledge without superstition or guesswork. It may not be known except through revelation how the law works, but experience teaches that it works relative to what is done for the body. When we learn how to behave in regard to our health and refuse to live correctly by this understanding, we find ourselves in the category of the stupid.

Gibby said:

Intelligence is the ability to discover and accurately interpret truth, compelled with the capacity to accept it and consistently apply it to daily living.

There are those who always live in this category because they learn not by their mistakes and are either contemptuous of law and order or are so weak as to be persuaded and influenced by others who have convinced themselves without reason

Society, leaders, family members, big money interests, and social pressures may encourage or impede health because the majority of people are like sheep – followers, like the sheep, unable to find their way alone. This is why Jesus likened man to sheep. The sheep is the only animal who by instinct cannot find its way home. Like sheep we need guidance, but we must still be the judge of what or whom we will follow. The inescapable fact is that the majority is always and has always been wrong and they become so, not on an individual basis, but because they follow the wrong leaders. Often the law is broken for the wrong reasons.

Gibby said:

Many of us live far below the character standards we are capable of achieving, simply because we fear the criticism or crave the approval of those among whom we

work and live. But never allow such lack of approval to keep you from high resolve or noble deed, for even a fool does not respect the fool.

As changes take place when a person begins to do even one thing in his favor, such as taking so simple a thing as slippery elm for an ulcer, the vast and wonderful possibilities reveal themselves if the whole law were understood and lived. Broken law exacts its final penalty like repentance. It does not take as long for nature to reward the body with health is it took to become sick. As soon as a beginning is made, the law becomes effective, working favorably in our behalf. When these laws are lived, restoration of health becomes an almost magical experience. When iridology is understood wonderful changes take place not only in our bodies but in our eyes. The iris is the nerve organ in the body which is the most sensitive and highly developed. It can instantly receive messages from any part of the body, reflecting pathology or restoration to health. The nervous system reflects the situation to the brain, which in turn causes the same situation to then be recorded on the eye.

Making a correct choice which proves to be predictable at all times develops strength; and if it is a sidestep from the ebb and flow of humanity's erroneous ways, we find that we do not have to be so rigidly subservient to the way of the world. Each time we prove one of these choices to ourselves, whether it is confidence in answer to a prayer or overcoming a stomach ache by taking the right herb, we are a step closer to an intelligent independence of our own soul and body.

Gibby said:

Truth walks a straight and undeviating path and shows partiality to no man.

Following are the testimonies of a few brave souls – among the many – start and stop, slide back and go forward, in this process of self-discipline, who have persevered long enough to make some interesting changes in their bodies and their irises.

Tapeworm

After attending a class taught by Mrs. Griffin I saw my eyes reflected a body in need of cleansing, so I started last June on her mild food diet and herbs. Immediately I became sick and stayed sick for six weeks when I decided to let up on it for a while. I didn't know how ill I was at the time. Some lumps appeared, they turned out to be malignant. I wasn't shattered. I knew other people had conquered the same malady through natural ways. I searched for every natural way I could find. I was one of the lucky ones. I had already started on the mild foods diet – being already familiar with it made it easier. I had never quit taking the herbs. After the doctors diagnosis I started again on the mild food diet.

After I had been on the diet (and herbs) about one month, I passed some nodules with long black fingerlike things on it. Odd looking, but the pathology report was negative, only mucus clumps. From that time to this (two months later) mucus has been passing out of my body. Then to my absolute horror, two days ago, I passed a tapeworm. That was enough for me, I wanted everything to shape up right now, but nature doesn't work that way. I can see by my eyes I have a way to go yet, before I have a completely clean intestinal tract. The path is before me, just wish I could travel it faster.

I love the Lord. He is my "guider". He has led me to the ways of truth and light. His is the credit and the glory and may he bless those who have the courage to stand, and especially those who stand and help others.

Theora Sheets

I would like to give my testimony to the effectiveness of LaDean Griffin's program of health. For the past three years I have been on mild food and the healing herbs that she describes in her book, *Is Any Sick Among You?*. This has been a very, very choice experience for me and a very spiritual one because at the time that I began this program, I was very ill. The medical Doctor – my gynecologist – had made tests with the pap smear and had indicated that I should have a hysterectomy because there were so many places where all the tissue was so poor and the threat of cancer was there. There were – I don't know exactly how they count these things – but they talked about how the count was lymph high and that it was indicated that I should have a hysterectomy and do some testing. I went in at that time and did have a D&C and they came up with the thought that I should wait a little while and see how things went. At that time my husband was very ill with cancer and I didn't feel that I could spend time in the hospital with him so sick and I pleaded with the doctors to let me wait until he was better before I had a hysterectomy.

I also had many other health problems. I had had inner ear troubles for years, and I would lose my equilibrium. I would lose my hearing and would be very ill with that problem. I also had a very severe back problem. I was seeing a chiropractor periodically, and getting slight results because of this, but it was not a true healing. It was only a sort of a pacifying thing that would ease the pain in my back and leg. I was unable to even get in and out of the car without having to lift my leg in and out. I was losing control over the muscles in that leg.

I began this program and stayed on it faithfully using the mild foods and the herbs. Immediately, my health began to improve and I began feeling better. The healing crises have been disturbing and upsetting because you feel that you are going back into the sickness again as your body tends to throw off the waste. But I have waded through the healing crises and I have always come up feeling better after I finished.

The doctors have made test, of course, since I have been very careful to get the tests every six months to check to see if there was any more cancer – any more problems there, and they have found nothing. In fact, two weeks ago when I went in for a checkup, the doctor said that he just couldn't believe how well my body has healed and how healthy the tissue is. I've also had heart problems in the past that have caused me lots of discomfort and have kept me from doing things that I enjoy doing and now at the present time I am working full-time. I'm very well. My heart never gives me any trouble and I don't have trouble with my back at all. My chiropractor has released me. He has shown me the x-rays that he has taken compared to the ones he took on me three years ago and he said, "I can't believe the improvement you have made in your bone structure and your bone quality." He said that "this shows that you are progressing in your health, rather than deteriorating." I am now age 55 and I feel better than I did when I was 35. My mind is clear and sharp and I am active and I love to be with people and share my feelings about this beautiful method of staying well and getting well. I might also say that I have had arthritis in the past, however, since I've been on the program it has gradually left me. I still have a few little nodules on my fingers, but I never have any pain from them in their gradually getting smaller and going away. This is a beautiful program of health and it has not kept me away from the doctor's office. I have continued to be checked and to have the tests made that are necessary to know what is going on and I have been thrilled to see the improvement that I have made and the doctors have been thrilled with that also. I think that it is important to watch what is happening when you started a program like this and continue to keep track of your health and improvement that is made. Good health is important to all of us, and it's important for us to know our bodies, to know the foods and herbs that are needed in our bodies to heal them when we're sick. I'm grateful for the knowledge that I have gained as I've worked on this program. It has been an inspiration to me to help me to improve my health and to live here upon this earth in joy and happiness and being able to help others. I am Theora Sheets and I'm happy to give my testimony to the truthfulness of this book and the great help that it is to those that read it and enjoy it and learn to live with what is given there as a way to find a better way of life.

Gary Gillum - see picture page 47

"The Staff of Life Overcomes the Staph of Job."

"Mirror, mirror on the wall, who's the fairest of them all?", quote I. " Certainly not a 'it's-just-caused-by-adolescence' pimply, 'it's-not-your-fault-you're-not Charles Atlas' skinny chassis such as yours," replied the reflection to me. With that outburst of subjective truth my frame fairly tensed with anger at my Jobian state, insomuch that I thought my bowel would straighten as a nail. (Sigh.) I guess I will have to outwait my adolescent years of pimple hood and awkwardness. But I am 24 years old now! And what do I have to show for it but horrid reminiscences of taxing dermatologists who froze, relaxed, drugged and wrapped my face, clearly silly, phisohexian hocus-pocus soaps and cold-then-hot-water-should-do methods to embattle my pores still further? (I was told chocolate caused my condition, but I didn't like chocolate.) What to show except for a missing appendix, whose 22 years were exhausted as a savior, along with staphylococcus bacteria, in releasing poisons from my warring frame. These conditions, of course, were caused by the medicians' brews in hospitals and campus health centers where the 'modern' priestcraft of medical malpractice flourished as did Baal in the days of Elijah three years following the mirror incidents, the lowly, mistreated, misunderstood but beautiful and delicious dandelion became an instrument in opening my eyes and set the stage for a meeting with LaDean. (Thenceforward my wife and I have annually celebrated that momentous occasion with wilted dandelions from our lawn.) It was not merely the word-of-mouth advertising which sent us to this remarkable woman, but the desire on the part of my wife and I to search for light and knowledge, especially since my graying skin condition dictated that we would try anything once to prevent my permanent mortification. After several visits with LaDean, she informed us that on my first visit she had felt that I might not make it. But I had followed her teaching as well as the promptings of the Spirit and soon found the way towards better health. (Even as I write these words I can feel miraculous changes within my body, changes which are quickening my body, my spirit, and my long-lost self-confidence. In the beginning it was necessary to rid my body of those creatures who fed upon my innards parasitically, and as months passed I fondly referred to them as Max, Maxine and the Maxmillions. Well, they have since departed this life with the aid of herbs, which possess one thing medical drugs lack – innate spirit. (Man cannot synthesize the spirit of an element or being, even if it is possible to duplicate physical and outward features.) A famous Mormon lawyer and Church leader, J. Reuben Clark, Jr. once speculated that the administration of the sick by the elders of the Church (James 5:14) is necessary in many cases of illness since the body's healing mechanisms had not learned all of the disease ridding functions while in its earlier estate. In addition, I personally believe that herbs provide an added intelligence to the body cells, training the individual cells and organs to slough off the poisons and bacteria and fight with renewed vigor. Not that the herb itself has no intrinsic medicinal value. On the contrary, its purpose is twofold, for Peter the Apostle had not only ordered the crippled man to arise, but offered his own assistance by giving him a hand. An example might illustrate this: the psyllium seed which helped my colon slough off and eliminate an 18 inch tumor definitely assisted. (That tumor I should also have immortalized in glass and formaldehyde only after I had allowed medical scientists to scrutinize it and wonder how I could have gotten it out except by the edge of a knife.) The cleaning of my pancreas by herbs was a most important aspect of my experience. But that process, even more so than that of ridding the body of parasites, depended equally on correct nutrition. The only 'nutrition' I had previously followed as the world's estimate of a balanced diet for a 'skinny toothpick' plus the opposite of a weight reducing formula: a fatty formula, consisting of double portions of meat, fats and carbohydrates, three meals per day during my college years. Well, we all know that stuffing elephantine amounts of 'food' into an Ichabod Cranian body does nothing for the glandular imbalance of the system except worsen the condition and throw the body into an metabolic tailspin toward an early transition. Upon beginning a correct diet for my own body, I recognized that throughout my years of adolescence I had suffered from migraine headaches, lack of energy, boils, hemorrhoids, and beginnings of stomach ulcers. It would take some time to alleviate entirely these sufferings. I lacked the sufficient energy in the beginning to go completely on a mucusless diet, so it was supplemented with goats milk and plenty of baked potatoes, which I grew to love. Several years later, I find that my favorite foods are fruits, nuts and seeds, and these provide me with all the taste bud enjoyment and energy I could ever have hoped for. True, I weigh no more, but the other diet had not solve the problem either. The important thing now is being rid of disease almost entirely. Decayed animal matter, cooked foods, and un-assimilatable substances could hardly feed a compost pile, let alone a human body.

I could recite numerous incidents which proved to me that I have found light and truth in the way I now live, but I will let the reader rest after a few choice ones: 1) A two-week cherry fast last summer found 2 tablespoons of mucus coming forth out of my sinuses, unaccompanied by any cold pain except the welcome pain of matter breaking loose in the head area. 2) While taking black walnut to extradite Max and his family of parasites, I felt the most angry rebellion ever in my lower bowel, and I felt it necessary to thank my large intestine, my heart and my other organs for the valiant battle they fought and won. 3) This past summer I experienced my first five day lemon and honey fast. I hungered for no other foods and possessed an over abundance of energy I previously had rarely – if ever – experienced. Utilizing the scientific method or reason is no precise method in determining the truth of anything, except temporarily. Only personal revelation and direction through the Spirit, providing the patient is teachable, is an eternal measure of eternal truths. Then the person will be able to discern his way through the temptations, quackery's, misconceptions and evil teachings of a world whose God is Mammon, and whose goal is to imprison mankind in darkness. The result for anyone who perseveres will be a pure and holy Temple fit for the permanent habitation of the Spirit while he yet lives, possessing not only a joyful, selfish life, but a happifying, selfless life of service to others. Who can think of a more wonderful blessing than that? I offer my thanks to she who offered her knowledge, wisdom and service in the face of blind persecution from those who are 'learned'.

The following herbs, along with a mucusless diet, enabled me to help my body (and will in the future help my body) to become healthier and clean itself of a pre-diabetic condition (cleansing of the pancreas), headaches, hemorrhoids and anemia:

Goldenseal (1/4 teaspoon three times per day)
Cayenne pepper
Lower bowel herb
Herbal pumpkin (4 tablets per day)
Liptrophic adjunct (2 per day)
Additional herbs and vitamins depending on condition, season and diet.

Today for a general cleansing of the body, which will someday bring me to perfect health I take the following herbs and vitamins:

Goldenseal (1/4 teaspoon three times per day)
Cayenne pepper

CS Formula
Nervine
Herbal pumpkin (6 tables per day)
Vitamin E and Vitamin B12 (one each per day)
Lecithin granules
Additional herbs and vitamins depending on condition. During the summer months I eat liberal amounts of sunflower seeds and exercise my neck twice daily in order to improve my eyesight. At present I need glasses only for driving. I used to wear them constantly.

Pumpkin seeds (as an aid to herbal pumpkin)
Fresh fruit (almost exclusively this summer)

Jeannine McKenzie - see picture page 47

I started on the mild foods in August, and I stayed on it very strictly without any deviation at all for about 3 1/2 months without anything else. The only herbs that I took at this time were licorice and some nervine herbs once in a while but not regularly, and the thing that I noticed the most, was that previous to this, I had really had problems with my hips. I could hardly walk up and down the stairs or do anything after just two or three hours of even mild work in my home. After this period of time, I could work from early in the morning – five and 6 o'clock till clear into the middle of the night without ever having this problem again. It never bothers me. This and just being able to get out of bed in the morning and not having that tired, tired feeling, which I'm sure came from the consumption of too much sugar and this type of thing. And how do I feel right now? I feel great! I'm taking other herbs and things now. I'm still on the mild foods, and I've added quite a lot of alfalfa, my glands, and more of the nervine herbs because I realize that this is what I need, and as I go along, this nervous, uncontrollable urge to just get out and away from things and not do the things I know I'm supposed to, is gone. It's really been wonderful. I lost 30 pounds.

Michael Tracy - see picture page 47

All too often, we tend to blame God for death, disease, and anything that goes wrong in our lives. This is, of course, both unfair and unreasonable. "It was never the intention, nor in the plan of God to produce disease, but as a logical consequence, thru disobedience of the divine laws of life, disease is produced." (*The Mucusless Diet Healing System*, Ehret, pg. 85)

We are, then, largely responsible for our own physical well-being, and there is no doubt in my mind that each of us will be held accountable for the manner in which we take care of our bodies.

I believe now is the time to learn and live the true laws of health, endeavoring to recall from antiquity the precious knowledge that was once held sacred by our biblical ancestors concerning these things. I believe that man can and will, with the help of the Lord, progress to the point where he will no longer be a slave to poor health. And I feel certain that these things will be accomplished with proper diet, herbs, and the work and inspiration the Restored Priesthood.

Because of the Mild Food Diet, and the judicious use of herbs, my wife and I have taken long strides in improving our health. For us, this new, exciting way of life has given us a feeling of vibrant rejuvenation and well-being. We know that it has strengthened us spiritually as well as physically. We are grateful that we have learned these things while still young and we are certain that the children that will be born to us will reap many benefits because of our diligence.

Yes, there have been a few times when we wanted to "cheat" on the diet. More than once I have seen a steaming rib roast, a Dairy Queen, or a Cheese Whistle that looked appealing. Nonetheless, the rewards received for avoiding these things are spectacular and well worth the effort involved in cultivating self-discipline.

My wife and I look and feel younger. Our eyes have become brighter and clearer, and our strength and stamina have increased. We share a firm belief that our efforts are purposeful and in keeping with sound religious teachings. We have a strong testimony of the truthfulness of the Mild Food Diet, and we know that anyone who adheres to it will enjoy the same benefits and blessings that have come to us.

Alexandra (Lexie) Veranth Harris

Today, I am a happy, healthy, slim, 34-year-old wife and mother of four children, counting our foster daughter. It was not always so!

It is my testimony that I have been to hell and back. I attribute my present happy state of affairs to prayer, the influence of the Holy Ghost testifying to me the truth of the diet as a higher law of eating so that I had the faith to stick it out when it took courage; and, to my loving, giving, understanding husband who would cook his own meat meals and supported me during my journey to health. He could so easily have made it harder on me or tried to make me feel guilty. At first I didn't have the willpower to cook and look at meat and bread dishes without eating them. I do now.

From infancy I have had what was diagnosed as chronic atrophic pyelonephritis. Which means I had one kidney stunted and atrophied from chronic infections. From two years before my first marriage and continuing through the 10 years of its duration I was plagued with constant chronic kidney and bladder infections which at times caused such pain that I required hospitalization. During the rest of the time the infections were controlled by strong antibiotics and almost constant pain pills and narcotics from percodan to morphine. During my first marriage my husband poured literally thousands of dollars into doctor and hospital bills. And countless more into pills of all kinds. I had major surgery three times. Minor surgery four or five times. Hospitalizations excepting the above at least once a year. And I even sought psychological help because of my misery and inability to care for my family. I learned that anyone who is that sick with a family to care for and no hired help or consistent help is bound to go a little balmy upstairs. I spent quite a few hours depressed and many nights sobbing into my pillow begging our Father in Heaven to help me out of my seemingly inescapable pit, as the doctors had said there was no known cure for chronic disease of my type.

I bore three children, two of whom were born with hyaline membrane disease, six weeks prematurely. The youngest required hernia surgery at three months. They both suffered chronic severe constipation from toddler age until we went on the diet a year ago when they were seven and eight years old respectively.

Almost 6 years ago I was converted to the Church of Jesus Christ of Latter-day Saints; and that is when my life made a drastic and steady change for the better. I stopped drinking and smoking. Became pregnant with my third child who was born normally; but with bad colic. At that time I received my Patriarchal blessing in which I was cautioned to be careful of the things regarding my health so that I would have vigor of body and mind. This was a new concept for me as I had always gone faithfully to the doctor and been an obedient patient. Then my baby came down with diarrhea for five or more weeks straight and the doctor couldn't stop it. That's when I visited my first health food store and my blessing began to make more sense to me. I began to see the vision of health. I took a health and nutrition class and read everything Adelle Davis wrote and anything else I could get my hands on.

At this point I should mention that, at the time of my marriage I was a Seattle Seafair Princess and was blessed with a very nice figure. Well, disease, drugs, four pregnancies and my delicious, gourmet and pastry cooking had ruined it. I'm 5'6" and with my bone structure should weigh around 114 pounds. During my years of sickness, I weighed from 130 to 145 pounds. After my third child, the first I had been able to nurse, I reasoned that since chocolate is bad for a nursing baby (I was a chocoholic) and a milk drinking mother was good for one, I would kill two birds with one stone and eat ice cream. That would satisfy my sweet craving (a lifelong urge) and we'd all be happy. The day came I weighed 175 pounds and no end in sight. I was into Adelle Davis at the time and threw out all canned, packaged and frozen foods; and ate a highly superior form of the great American diet. I began baking my own bread and switched to goats milk. My children still suffered from constipation which was a nightmare; but my weight over a period of two years gradually decreased until I stabilized at 145 pounds. I felt better because I looked better and was proud of myself. However, we were still sick, although not as drastically.

Then the children and I moved to Seattle. Now cooking to please myself, I cut out most meat and most sweets from the diet. At this time, I experienced my first great cleansing crisis, pneumonia; although at the time I didn't realize it. My dear mother nursed me to health and then we moved to Provo, Utah, where I had the good fortune to move in across the street from my future husband and next door to Gary and Lyn Gillum.

I had had the feeling deep down for several months that I should try vegetarianism; but the whole subject baffled and scared me. I had been raised closely associated with the medical profession both in my immediate family and as employers and had quite a knowledge of medicine both as a matter of curiosity and as a sympathetic viewer of the doctors often times selfless and dedicated role. And through my studies I had been scared by nutritionists claims of the deleterious effects of strict vegetarianism. My curiosity and desire for truth led me to ask my neighbors about their way of eating as I had heard some pretty interesting remarks from acquaintances. The first thing they told me was about the delicious pizza they had made the night before with potatoes. All sorts of crazy scenes passed thru my mind. Then they acquainted me with LaDean's works. I read her book and knew by the burning and recognition of truth inside me that what LaDean wrote about with a higher law of eating. It made intellectual sense. It supplied the missing pieces in my jigsaw puzzle of knowledge about health and diet. I decided to try it; but put off following it strictly until after my impending honeymoon. I just couldn't see passing up all those fantastic Chinese restaurants and lobster dinners and fine pastries on my honeymoon. Well, you guessed! On the fifth day of my honeymoon (we took it with the kids) I ended up in Heber city hospital hobbling from bathroom to emergency room and biting my lips in pain. From then on pain dictated my actions. I couldn't see repeating the endless expensive cycle of drugs and doctors with no cure in sight. So I threw away the hospital pills and went on to fruits and vegetables, a few nuts and seeds, some raw juice and herbs for the bladder and kidneys. I took catnip for my nerves, goldenseal and licorice root for my kidneys and for my craving for sweets. CS to cleanse my system, psyllium seed powder mixed with juice for my bowels (which were in horrible shape) and I fasted and prayed a lot. I slowly got better. I would have improved faster, but I had a hang-up about taking enemas. One day after coming off a 14 day fast my tummy swelled like I was six months pregnant within three days after I resumed eating. I forced myself to take an enema and the pain and swelling subsided within the hour. I discovered that poisons will pass into the bladder from a toxic colon. I have since been concentrating on strengthening my bowels. I now consider myself healed of my main pain causing problems; but have a way to go, before completely healing all of the organs in areas of my body that were almost destroyed by drugs and faulty diet. I have my teenage figure back and look about 10 to 15 years younger than I did at my worst. During the period of my greatest cleansing I appeared skinny and haggard to others, even though I had progressed far enough to have conquered the pain. But continuing the same diet of fruits, vegetables, nuts, seeds, a small amount of raw honey and juices I gradually gained back a small amount of weight to what is normal for me and gained energy and color. The only dietary change I underwent was to switch from cooked to raw vegetables, shredded and added to salads and an increase in herbs. And more regular enemas, of course. I also now try to drink at least two quarts of carrot juice and other fresh raw fruit and vegetable juices each day to build up my body nutrition. I've thrown out most of my supplements, retaining vitamin C and E, and maybe garlic pills. I used to spend a fortune on food supplements after I threw out the prescribed medicine. Now I use juices and herbs to cleanse and heal. Lately I have used the skinny formula, which has produced the most terrific head cleansing and pouring forth of mucus I would not have believed possible. I have had iridology pictures taken, but my body was so deteriorated that I saw only slight improvement. If I had had recent pictures however you would notice that my eyes have turned from what people saw as a darkish gray but mistook often for brown, to a much lighter blue with heavy white acute healing lines. In every area where there was a black closed lesion there is a thick mass of healing lines.

During my illness, and cleansing, healing, change of diet, I made the mistake of worrying my family long distance by telling them what I was and wasn't eating and how wonderfully skinny I was getting. Then six months ago we were able to visit. You can imagine my great feeling of exultation as I saw their eyes light up in delighted surprise and heard their remarks of approval and curiosity. Then just after Christmas my mom, Ruth Veranth called and asked me to visit and teach her the diet. I went armed with the LaDean's books, some herbal formulas, an iridology chart and the determination to buy her a juicer. I bear my testimony that our Father answered my prayers and if the most famous credentialed doctor in the world told me I was wrong or if the powers that be all rallied against it I would not change my way of eating and herbing, as my children and I suffered hell with our bodies and now know budding health and have happiness.

The following is a poem my mother woke up with on her mind one morning while I was teaching her the program.

Here's to tricks in '76

No more will the bod be a jinx.
'Twill look and feel like a merry minx.
Joy and laughter will erase the kinks,
Charles and I out to the links,
And no more garbage to make us finks,
Eat it and the whole world shrinks,
And a house full of junk saps the energy methinks.
To the depths of despair the weary one sinks.
Careful now – trim your wicks.
Here's to celestial heights in '76!

Ruth Veranth

It is with pure joy that I offer my testimonial on the efficacy of LaDean's nutritional "way of life." Since my daughter, Lexie, brought me to the knowledge six weeks ago I've shed 20 pounds, and have never felt more buoyant, energetic, free and alive than with my newfound delicious diet of live fruit, vegetables, herbs, nuts and seeds. Dramatically, unhealthy cravings and leg muscle cramps disappeared as if by magic. I want to shout my praises to the house tops; my friends are amazed and ask for this pragmatic answer to one of life's most important problems – how to eat right and greet each new day – with sparkling enthusiasm, brimming over with energy and happiness.

Wyonna Kruse

Something was wrong! I was so tired all the time, with a shaky feeling inside. At times my body appeared to be going 100 miles an hour, and I felt I had to get food inside of me to slow this down. This extreme tired feeling persisted and I kept tuning it out. My husband was experiencing extreme physical problems, and I knew this was not the time or place for me to be getting sick. At the insistence of a friend, I went to a doctor.

The usual tests and x-rays were done. I took huge amounts of protein to build my adrenaline. I began swelling and I experienced so much bloating when I ate, that I had to take chewable enzymes. My daily intake of hormone pills and thyroid was astounding. I had learned to check my vitamins for purity from coal tar, and I knew they were not causing my discomfort. (Incidentally, should you be interested in your own vitamins, place the vitamin in an old spoon, heat from a lighted candle turns it black, if they are made from coal tar. Vitamin showing this coloring should be dumped.)

Time passed. I went again to the doctor. I showed a very high glucose test shooting up to 480 and then dropping to 47. My doctor showed me the blood tests under the microscope. When he pointed out the little globules moving so sparkly in my bloodstream, I asked him, "Are these cancer cells?" He evaded my question indirectly by saying, "You do have a bad infection in your blood." He gave me a prescription for several drugs and one potent antibiotic. None of these drugs appeared to be helping my condition. My doctor made a serum from my urine, which I took twice each week. Nothing helped. Then I heard about the book, *Is Any Sick Among You?*

I began attending the classes on iridology. When I saw my own eyes, I realized that I was much worse off than my husband, who had suffered a coronary. I knew that I had a strong inherent body and with the help of the Lord, and my family and friends, I could discipline myself to get on this cleansing program and stay on it.

176

Those who have been on the program know that when you first begin the routine, you clean so fast that the toxic waste moves into your bloodstream and makes you deathly ill.

I hadn't eaten much this day and about dinnertime I began noticing terrible pains. I had committed myself to attend a meeting this evening. While sitting in this meeting I experienced such terrible pains, severe like labor pains only they were in my liver and pancreas regions. I could time their occurrence and reoccurrence just like labor pains. I was almost out of my mind with pain. I had to be excused from the meeting. I didn't want to call the doctor and I had to get relief, so I took a coffee enema. (Coffee stimulates the liver) I took a quart of water, but I couldn't expel it. Nothing would come out. For 30 minutes I massaged and worked my colon. I rolled on the floor, I walked, I tried different positions. The pain was still intense, but not as intense as before I put the water in. I took another quart of the water and it was at least 15 minutes later that I was able to expel the water with a large clump or mass. I should have had this mass checked. I'll always believe that it was a tumor that had passed from my body.

Herbs will loosen and pull the waste from the intestines. The intestines are like a sink, they can become plugged up. We wonder how they can become so plugged up. This is what had been happening to me. I had been pulling all this waste matter from my intestines which caused this intense pain. People who have been on Laetrile (apricot seed) and chaparral herb, over a period of time, will experience this intense pulling as the fecal loosens from the body. The pulling become so great that it appears to cause a bloated feeling and you wish you could take a knife and "stick" yourself as the farmers did their cows in the years back.

My purpose in taking time to write how I feel physically, is for you readers to realize the urgency to get on this program, if you are having problems. I was thrilled with my doctor's last report. My protein was higher than it has ever been and my hypoglycemia is much better.

I have noticed that people will give up anything but their food, and the food habits they enjoy. Usually it takes a real live "jolt", mine was "terminal disease" to push one on the program. Self-discipline is the key to the program, through the years we rely so much on the arm of flesh. I keep telling myself that I have to stay on the program – plan certain days for the cleansing process with herbs and then follow-up with a strict diet of mild foods. The toxic in my body has to be released for me to get completely well. I have had to learn to live each day as the sun comes up. Some days my mind wants to go, but I have difficulty dragging my body along. Without my work, I'd give up. The Lord works in a mysterious way – maybe this is the reason he is teaching me to discipline myself. I have learned to say, "I'm not on a diet, I have low blood sugar and I eat mild foods." I am feeling much better now than I have felt for so long that I can't believe one can feel this good and still be not well. I didn't get this disease overnight. My body has probably been working on this for 30 years.

Don't let anyone tell you this is an easy program to follow. There are good days and days that are bad, but as Abraham Lincoln stated so beautifully, "God is the silent partner in all great enterprises,"... And I have gained an inner strength and peace of mind by placing my burdens on Him.

From the pen of the poet, Phillips Brooks, "O my young friends, the world is beautiful and... Life is full of purpose."

Wouldn't I be robbing God if I were to give less than my very best to the program?

CHAPTER 5

TO STAND ALONE

The Lord has told us to become as a little child in order to enter the Kingdom of Heaven. The trust and love of a child, even in a parent not worthy of that trust, is a beautiful thing. Is this the childlike attribute He was talking about? Can a childlike trust in God be represented continually as a way of life? Too much time is spent in trusting in the arm of flesh and not enough in trusting God. We lean so heavily upon each other that we miss the opportunity of direct contact with a higher power. The conflict of trusting in the arm of flesh when everyone is so self-seeking, leaves little room for inner rebuilding of the soul. Unique individuality and intense spiritual power must first be achieved alone, away from the crutch and weaknesses of other people.

Maturation depends upon mother and dad; but even though we then begin to fly alone we still need guideposts to follow. Because we have had little training in these new pursuits, we either muddle along making all the mistakes humanity is capable of making, or we wisely seek the eternal wisdom of the Scriptures and great minds of the past to discover what standards were upheld in their way of life. As these guideposts dot the landscape of our world, eternal trust is discovered. It then takes form and correct pattern is recognized, a definite procedure that must be observed in order to find man's most sought after prize – joy. Joy follows good health, but in order to have good health we must use wisdom. To acquire wisdom, we must learn either by trial and error or by studying the past mistakes of others.

As the complex problems of making a living and raising a family begin to crowd in upon us, we are often persuaded and influenced from all sides to make the incorrect decision. Before we can stand with God we must be able to stand alone, away from the opinions of others, away from leaning on other people. This is what is called courage. Would we be happy with our adult children if they came home every day for us to tie their shoes, or to ask is to do any of the things an adult is supposed to be capable of doing alone? By the same token, there are things we must learn to do by way of making certain judgments and choices which would be as bothersome to the Lord as if we had asked him to come down and tire our shoes every day. Some people have the idea that they must ask God to make all of their decisions for them and they call this faith. Somewhere along the way we must learn what God's laws require and make plans to stay within those boundaries. When I think of how honest and just a man my father was, I remember before I did anything questionable or wrong that I would ask what my dad would have done or thought.

When my dad was asked to take a high-paying job as a radio announcer and refused the position, I said to him, "I'll bet I know why you didn't take the job. You have always said radio announcers were liars, advertising obnoxious products detrimental to health." He said, "That's right, I could not advertise cigarettes, beer or even foodless food sprinkled with sugar, and tell children these foods would make them strong." Everyone has not had the example of goodly parents but we **do** have the example of great minds, prophets and Scriptures to light our path.

There is a great difference between being completely dependent on the Lord, completely subservient, completely loving and completely childlike than not being able to make any decisive choice or sacrifice. The Lord placed a head upon our shoulders with the body attached and forced us to do only one thing: **choose**. It has been regularly said by Edward Young, the English poet of the 16th century:

On the soft bit of luxury most kingdoms have expired.

If God made all of our decisions we would always make the right decision. Therefore we would be like a robot, without learning in the final analysis, why God's way is best. The Talmud makes a significant observation:

> *The best preacher is the heart*
> *the best teacher is time*
> *the best book is the world*
> *the best friend is God.*

To teach us the truth about pleasure and pain, Pope the English author said:

> *Reasons whole pleasure, all the joys of sense,*
> *lie in the words health, peace, and competence.*

What great rewards there are in accomplishment of making the right choice and of doing something well. Robert Louis Stevenson said:

> *He has achieved success who has lived well,*
> *laughed often and loved much; who has gained*
> *the respect of intelligent men and the love*
> *of little children; who has filled his niche*
> *and accomplished his task; who has left the*
> *world better than he found it, whether by an*
> *improved poppy, a perfect poem, or a rescued soul;*
> *who has never lacked appreciation of*
> *earth's beauties nor failed to express it;*
> *who has always looked for the best in others*
> *and given the best he has; whose life is an*
> *inspiration, whose memory, a benediction.*

Real joy is found in obedience to the law in common and ordinary things. A mother's domain is a palace filled with ordinary things where all the normal necessary desires are gratified: the table, the bath, a clean, comfortable bed, the laundry. This beauty and refuge from the world is the home, which she creates for her family. S. J. Hail said:

We need not power or splendor, wide halls or lordly dome! The good, the true, the tender, these form the wealth of home.

For the father, joy is also found in the ordinary. Lord Houghton said:

Do not grasp at the starts, but do life's plain common work, as it becomes certain that daily duties and daily bread are the sweetest things in life

Plutarch, scholarly historian of the Greeks, said:

That state of life's most happy where superfluities are not required and necessities are not wanting.

The satisfaction of winning the security for his family by the sweat of his brow – knowing he is the provider, teacher and protector of his family – brings joy and splendor to manhood. Plutarch reflects in his historical writings:

The man who first brought ruin upon the Roman people was he who pampered them by largesses and amusements.

Seneca, the Roman statesman, said

Great is he who enjoys his earthenware as if it were plate, and not less great is the man to whom all plate is not more than earthenware.

Rousseau, the French philosopher, said:

Temperance and labor are the two best physicians of man; labor sharpens the appetite and temperance prevents from indulging to excess.

Socrates, wisest of the Greeks, said:

Contentment is natural wealth,

Luxury, artificial poverty.

Great men of the past have recorded their findings in decisive language to light our path if we but search and find. Cervantes defined Proverbs as short sentences drawn from long experience. These philosophies, with their old familiar road signs, seem to appear in all languages and for all people as the infallible laws to happiness. Horace Greeley said:

The darkest hour in any man's life is when he sits down to plan how to get money without earning it.

J. M. Gibby said:

Iniquity creepeth in wherever selfishness, pride and haughtiness unlock the door.

Solomon taught us:

Go to the art, thou sluggard; consider her ways and be wise; which having no guide, overseer or ruler, provideth her meat in summer, and gathereth her food in the harvest.

My dad used to say, but I do not know who wrote it:

It is following the path of least resistance that makes rivers and man crooked.

Goethe the poet said:

If you want to make life easy make it hard.

Shakespeare said:

There can be no better sign of a brave mind than a hard hand.

To conquer self is a part of the pathway to joy. Da Vinci said:

You will never have a greater or lesser dominion than that over yourself.

Aristotle said:

He overcomes a stout enemy who overcomes his own anger.

Solomon said:

Who then is free? The wise man who can govern himself.

Christ laid down the fundamental principles of self-discipline as He ended His Sermon on the Mount:

Enter ye in at the strait gate, for wide is the gate and broad is the way that leadeth to destruction and many there be which go in thereat; because strait is the gate and narrow the way which leadeth unto life, and few there be that find it.

When we find great, happy and successful men, we find men of noble purpose and high spirituality who follow a straight line to accomplishing a great task by setting righteous goals and aiming courageously toward them. Then when we seek to find health by leaving the rules we have brilliant words to light our path. Paul said:

Be not deceived; God is not mocked, for whatsoever a man soweth that shall he also reap. He that soweth to the flesh shall of the flesh reap corruption. He that soweth to the spirit shall of the spirit reap life everlasting.

Byron said:

Vice digs her own voluptuous tomb.

Channing said:

Sensuality is the grave of the soul.

Pliny said

Lust is an enemy to the purse, a food to the person, canker to the mind, a corrosive to the conscience, a weakness of the wit, a besotter of the senses, and finally a mortal bane to all the body.

Longfellow said:

The blossoms of passion, gay and luxuriant flowers, are bright and full of fragrance, but they beguile us and lead us astray and their odor is deadly.

Socrates said:

The end of life is to be like God and the soul following God will be like him.

Daniel Webster said:

A conscience void of offense before God and man is an inheritance for eternity.

J.M. Gibby said:

He achieves in vain who in the process does not develop sound character, only he who is constantly learning and serving has a truly abundant life.

The Psalmist wrote:

What is man, oh Lord, that thou art mindful of him, and the Son of Man that thou visitest him. For thou hast made him a little lower than the angels and hast crowned him with glory and honor. Thou madest him to have dominion over the works of thy hands; Thou hast put all things under his feet. Oh Lord, our Lord, how excellent is thy name in all the earth.

We need to rejoice that we have been fashioned so beautifully so as to have happiness and success through obedience to the law. Samuel said:

> *Behold, to obey is better than sacrifice and to hearken than the fat of rams.*

The beautiful words of the Lord to Joshua as he led his people into the land of promise, rings loud and clear – giving us hope and courage to go on:

> *Only be thou strong and of good courage; be not afraid, neither be thou dismayed; for the eternal is with thee, whithersoever thou goeth.*

I have touched only upon a few of the great writings of the past, with the hope that our horizons may have broadened, that we have emerged from their words, realizing that life is a beautiful experience and that when we seek to watch for the road signs – yet standing on our own feet, building ever building courage, goodness, and beauty into our lives – we will not be easily turned aside by evil and designing men in the last days. We will not allow someone else to make such serious decisions concerning our health nor to our freedom of choice.

Some so-called experts in the field of medicine, who are still standing on the intellectual premise that the next few years will be an immunological period are even looking forward to transplanting genes and scientifically make chemical changes in the molecule. They think they can stop manic-depressives and women outnumbering men. They call it genetic engineering but I call it "trying to play God." They failed to understand the principle that after curing a person of his mental or psychological problems he seems to be a carrier to his offspring and so doctors intend to immunize against such defects. Immunology defined is: the total means by which the organism defends itself against all foreign substance. Are we going to allow a few scientists to run us and our children on this gauntlet of rearranging our genes so they can swell with pride and say, "I made him what he is" – like a robot or a Frankenstein monster. Isn't it time we began to make these individual changes in our own lives and in our society? Isn't it time we recognized that science has far too long used us as the scapegoat in their endless pursuit to find answers so as to change the existing laws of heaven and earth rather than seeking to live by the laws that already exist? Isn't it time we improved upon these laws, living them to perfection, rather than trying to change them to suit someone's idea of how God should have made His world? We all know that great art re-creates realism in a perfect form. Why not make realism into a perfect form rather than like the art of Picasso and Rodin who have tried to change beauty into their own grotesque, senseless idea of what art should be.

God has told us:

> Be ye therefore perfect even as your Father in heaven is perfect.

Science has far too long looked for the answers in the wrong places when it comes to human life. Besides who is going to play God and pick and choose our genes – only these unsure, imperfect men who feed their egotistical minds with their own supremacy and intellectual superiority. Are we raising more Hitler's or are we merely worshiping science in the same way men of old worshipped the Golden calf.

Seven hundred years ago the church ignored Roger Bacon's plea for restraint. The myopia of the people who lived with superstition caused Roger Bacon to cry out for scientific study. He feared that their reliance on the church would keep them ignorant. We have another kind of myopia in our day and time when man has developed a blind, single-minded reliance, placing all his hope in future with science and so-called men of learning. Isn't it time for us to reevaluate the "old" laws of God and apply them today to our environment and our relationships with one another? Or would we prefer to become perfect people robots at the hands of a few so-called intellectuals?

The Scientist and Doctor have become the great High Priest – where medicine has become a religion. But like the 16th century church, medical science is going to have to brace itself for the

Reformation, because thinking people everywhere have become disenchanted and are looking for and finding alternative solutions to their problems. They are learning preventative medicine and discovering that they do not want this dictatorship protection of a science which holds a pistol to their head with the continual claim that it is good for them. Neither does modern man anymore want to be babysat by a dangerous maniac. Concerned men and women everywhere are going back to the old simple rules which God has set down and finding health and peace, as they learn to stand on their own feet, take care of their own bodies and in effect refuse to lean on the arm of flesh. There is great courage shown in the quiet consistence of well doing.

CHAPTER 6

TO WALK BY FAITH

It has often been said, "The eyes are the Windows of the soul." In these past chapters we observed that the eyes are the Windows of the body, but we must not forget that they are also a reflection of the soul or spirit. Personologists maintain that certain physical features of the eyes reflect certain personality traits. It is interesting that all feelings and emotions (according to personology) are located in and around the eye structures; for example, a person who is tolerant has a wide space between the eyes, an affectionate person has a large Iris. Analytical ability shows on the eyelids and a critical person has a downward slant to the outside of the outer canthus. How the eye is positioned in the socket tells us something else. When the eye is deep set, a person is thoughtful with many serious ideas; when it is not deep set the person has great drive. Humor is shown by the crows feet at the corners of the eyes. High-curved brows indicate dramatic flair; straight eyebrows show aesthetic traits. When the brows are straight and meet in the center, we have the artist. Sharp angular eyebrows show a good measurement ability, perception in mechanical judgment. When there is a good ability to use words the texture of the skin on the lower lids has pebble like or crisscross lines rather than smoothness. Good judgment shows up in the placement of the eyes, where the eyes are equally placed, with one neither higher or lower than the other.

Personologists also maintain that these features can change if the trait is recognized and there is sufficient desire to change. This desire stimulates the already computed habits to make a correction in personality. Like learning to drive, it takes continual conscious effort to make this change. As the change is occurring, the facial features reflect the trait being changed and adjust accordingly. Have you ever observed an elderly person who has lived a saintly life, whose beauty and softness seems to defy all description? Then have you also observed the person who has lived a life of sham, gradually developing an ugliness of soul, where features change, transforming not only physical features but reflecting the evil from within, out through the eyes? Evil or good reaches out from the Windows of the soul, and people quickly respond.

An evil look in the eyes, an empty look, a lonely look, a lost look, a weird look, and insane look, a weary look, a look of love, a look of pain, a kindly look, a look of gratitude, a generous look, a forgiving look, a tender look, an embarrassed look, a look of fear, a look of remorse, a look of joy, a look of grief or anger: all of these and more can be seen instantly reflecting outward from the eyes, from the soul and without words. These reflections are responded to by anyone within range, including our quiet, dumb friends of the animal world.

This reminds me of the time our big male collie dog was patiently allowing our recently weaned kittens to snuggle up to him and suck. As I came out the back door and saw with surprise what was going on, I said in a voice that could only have shamed him, "Pepper, for goodness sake, what are you doing?" He quickly shook them free, gave me an embarrassed look and walked slowly away with head down and tail between his legs. "The eyes are truly the Windows of the soul." Soul to soul through the eyes is one of the best means of communication with which we have been blessed.

It is with interest that we note the discoveries of great men who have pioneered the Bates method of eye exercise, who have learned that the shape of the eyeball is controlled by external muscles, which respond instantaneously to action, and that no refraction state, normal or abnormal, can be permanent. Consequently there are many things that enter into the ability to see well, and not all of these interferences with accurate site are by any means identified strictly with the body but must, by all logical reasoning, be associated also with the spirit within the body. You have heard it said, "I was so mad I couldn't see straight." Whether we realize it or not, all the things we feel, think and do have a definite effect on what we project out through the eyes as well as the color beauty of our auras.

I found a small scrap of paper among my dad's papers in his own handwriting which said:

May we always search for the good and beautiful, in living and good books, so that we might be better equipped to be of service to others.

A thing of beauty is considered to be a joy forever. There is nothing more beautiful than the reflection from the eyes and the aura of a great spirit, filled with an enthusiastic love of living and people.

If we would realize how often we are not a picture of beauty and not radiating forth from our inner soul those loving things that bless and bring joy to the beholder, we might learn to think more on a positive and righteous level.

Carlisle has left us a forceful paragraph to help us in our searching, that we might reach into more lofty realms:

He is of the earth, but his thoughts are with the stars. Mean and petty his wants and desires; yet they serve a soul exalted with glorious aims – with immortal longings – with thoughts which sweep the heavens and wander through eternity. A pigmy standing on the crest of this small planet, his far-reaching spirit stretches outward to the infinite, there alone finds rest.

Puny man in his reaches heavenward seems so small in the vast space of time and eternity, and yet Shakespeare wrote:

What a piece of work is man; how noble in reason! How infinite in faculties! In form and moving, how express and admirable! In action how like an angel! In apprehension, how like God!

Emerson gave us a lovely thought:

As much of heaven is visible as we have eyes to see.

It is not how much we can see but rather what can we contribute to beauty in the sight of others that is important. How can we be a light in the darkness so that this darkness might flee from us as well?

Helen Keller, who lived in darkness, has beautifully said:

There is no lovelier way to thank God for your sight than by giving a helping hand to someone in the dark.

When we have learned the truth do we share it? When we have had a spiritual testimony do we hide it away and forget it? Are we like the ship's captain who, in a bad storm, began to pray," Dear God, I haven't called upon you for 15 years and if you will save me now I won't bother you for another 15 years." Can we learn to pray always, not in a bothersome way, but rather with gratitude and hope? Can we stand on her own feet and yet trust that all things are done for our best good? Can we learn the laws of God and seek to obey them without being bitter about those laws, wishing it was some other way we might devise? The apostle Paul said:

Love worketh no ill to his neighbor: therefore love is the fulfilling of the law.

Love is the beginning of faith, the reaching out in trust to that God who created all the wonder and glory that is life on earth. Mark remembers a promise of the master:

Therefore I say unto you what things so ever ye desire, when he pray, believe that ye receive them, and ye shall have them.

In order to be in the company of God we must desire to be like Him, to obey Him in all things. Paul gave some excellent instruction to his brother and on how to become more God-like:

Finally, brethren whatsoever things are true, whatsoever things are honest, whatsoever things are just, whatsoever things are pure, whatsoever things are of good report, if there be any virtue and if there be any praise – think on these things.

Christ said:

Behold, I stand at the door and knock; if any man hear my voice and open the door, I will come in unto him and sup with him and he with me.

A spark from a fire will only rise to the extent that it reduces itself to flame – if there is any dirt on it, it will rise only feebly and the dirt on it will soon consume its flame and bring it back to the ground. Not unlike the flame is man. With the weight of dirt and dross clinging to him, his soul will rise upward only feebly.

If we wish to rise we must seek the good, the wise, the pure, the gentle, the kindly, the loving, the beautiful. Lincoln said:

Die when I may, I want it said of me by those who knew me best, that I always plucked a thistle and planted a flower wherever I thought a flower would grow.

In order to walk in faith and listen to that still small voice that whispers "all is well, you are here to learn my child and you are learning well, fear not for I walk beside you with love and tender concern" – we must live with lofty thoughts, high resolves, noble deeds, kind and loving thoughts, seeking after that which is good and pure light. Walt Whitman said:

Keep your face toward the sunshine and the shadows will fall behind you.

There is much in this world that is shoddy, filled with degradation, pain and sorrow because people seek after evil and in its discovery, reap the wrath of a just God upon their heads. There is a great difference between the wrath of God and the refiner's fire, and when we begin to live by the spiritual rather than by the sensual, we soon discover the difference. Paul understood the difference very well when he said:

By whom also we have access by faith into this grace wherein we stand, and rejoice in hope of the glory of God. And not only so, but we glory in tribulations also; knowing that tribulation worketh patience; and patience experience; and experience hope; and hope maketh not ashamed; because the love of God is shed abroad in our hearts by the Holy Ghost which is given unto us. (Romans 5:2)

May the love of life and God fill you with the beauty of spirit which sheds its light forth from your eyes and the glow of your aura – to enriching the lives of all you meet – is my prayer for you, that such lights may begin to glow in the darkness and fill the whole world with the warmth of heavenly light. May you have eternal part in such glory.

BIBLIOGRAPHY

Books:

Bates, W.H. *Better Eyesight Without Glasses*. New York: Holt, Reinhardt and Winston, Inc.

Bealle, Morris, *Dangerous Doses.* Washington, DC: Columbia Publishing Co.

Bealle, Morris, *Super Drug Story.* Washington, DC: Columbia Publishing Co.

Best and Taylor. *Psychological Basis Medical Practice.*

Boyd. *Textbook of Pathology.*

Breasted, J.H. Edwin Smith. *Surgical Papers.* Chicago: University of Chicago, 1930.

Christopher, Dr. *Herbal Manuscript.* Provo, Utah: Bi-World Publishing.

Coon, Nelson. *Using Wayside Plants.* New York: Hearthside Press, Inc.

Culpepper. *Culpepper's Complete Herbal.* London: W. Foulham & Co., LTD

Dawson, *Medicine in Ancient Egypt: Annals of Medical History. Vol. VI.* Encyclopedia Britannica, Library Research Service, 1924.

Ehret, Arnold. *Mucusless Diet Healing System.* Beaumont, California: Ehret Lit. Publishing Company

Forbes, Allen. *Our Garden Friends the Bugs*. New York: Exposition Press.

Gibby, J. Melvin, *Sand for the Rails.* Salt Lake City, Utah: Deseret Press.

Griffin, LaDean, *Herbs to the Rescue.* Provo, Utah: Bi-World Publishing.

Griffin, LaDean, *No Side Effects: The Return to Herbal Medicine.* Provo, Utah: Bi-World Publishing, 1975

Holy Bible, The, KJV

Howell. *Textbook of Physiology*

Gytcgebs, Alma R. *Indian Herbology North America.* Ontario, Canada: Marco

Illich, Ivan, Calder and Boyer. *Medical Menesis*

"Intestinal Parasites" Modern Medical Counselor, Chapter 42, Mountain View, California: Pacific Press Publishing Association.

Jensen, Bernard. *The Science and Practice of Iridology.* Solano Beach, California: Jensen Products and publishing.

Kadans, Joseph, *Modern Encyclopedia of Herbs.* West Nyack, New York: Parker Publishing Company, Inc.

Kirschner, H. E. *Nature's Healing Grasses.* Riverside, California: H.C. White Publishing Company, Inc.

Kloss, Jethro, *Back to Eden.* Coalmont, Tennessee: Longview Publishing House.

Kreig, Margret. *Green Medicine.*

Kreigg, Theodor, *Fundamental Basis of Iris Diagnosis.*

Kritzer, J. Haskel, *Testbook of Iridiagnosis.* Chicago: 1924

Livingston, Virginia, *Cancer: A New Breakthrough.*

Loewenfeld, Claire. *Herb Gardening.* London: Faber and Faber

Lucas, Richard. *Nature's Medicines.* New York: Awards Books.

Master Herbology. Ogden, Utah: Research Technical Service.

McCoy, Frank. *Fast Way to Health.* Los Angeles: McCoy Publishing Inc.

Meyer, Joseph. *The Herbalist.* Brand McNally Company – Conkey Division.

Netter, F *Volume of Medical Illustrations, Nervous System.*

Shohl. *Mineral Metabolism.*

Steiger, Brad, *Medicine Power.* Garden City, New York: Doubleday.

Taylor, Thomas. *Porphyry: On Abstinence from Animal Food.* Barnes & Noble, 1965.

Tobe, John. *Proven Herbal Remedies.* Canada: Provoker Press.

Vogel, Virgil J. *American Indian.* New York: Ballantine Books

Wigmore, Ann. *Why Suffer.* Boston: Rising Sun Christianity.

White, Ellen G. *The Ministry of Healing.* Mt. View, California: Pacific Press Publishing Association.

Young. *Handbook of Roentgen Diagnosis.*

Periodicals:

"DMSO Results Fantastic," Pleasanton, California, Herald and News, December 20, 1969.

Fredricks, Carlton. "Hotline to Health," Prevention Magazine, June, 1974

Helleboe, Herman E. "Recognition for Need to Prevent Sickness," American Journal of Public Health, May, 1971.

Knowles, John H. "The Coming Change in Medicine," Intellectual Digest, February, 1974.

Merrill, Joseph E. "Eat Flesh Sparingly," Address in Tabernacle, April 5, 1948

Mooney, Booth, "American people are eating more chemicals per capita than ever before," Plain Truth, February, 1970

National Observer, November 8, 1972

"Needless Surgery," National Observer, July 29, 1972

Smith, Tony, London Times, March 14, 1975

Stevens, Guy P. "Some Foods Are Drugged," The Improvement Era, March 1954

Sullivan, Bernice, "The Organic Conversion," San Francisco Examiner and Chronicle

INDEX

A

Acidophilus, 24, 61
Acne, 98
Acute Condition, 28, 36, 37
Adams, Loretta, 128
Addison's Disease, 30, 86, 110
Adrenal, 29
Adrenal Hormone, 32, 39
Alfalfa, 29
Allergies, 152
Aloe Vera, 85
Analgesia, 16
Anemia, 40, 66
Angina, 16, 21
Antibiotics, 71, 85, 86, 89, 90, 103, 106, 143, 169
Antidotes, 16
Anti-Inflammative, 16
Aristotle, 182
Arsenic, 41
Arteriosclerosis, 21
Arthritis, 16
Aspen Bark, 109
Assimilation, 31
Autonomic Wreath, 19, 22, 25, 28, 29, 35, 42

B

B Complex, 28, 29, 61, 85, 132, 139, 143, 144, 150, 153
Backache, 79
Bacon, Roger 185
Bayberry, 68
Beal, Linda 147
Biddulph, Karen 87
Biddulph, Kent 91
Birth Control, 93, 115

Black Cohosh, 30, 75, 102, 146
Black Cohosh, 30
Black Walnut, 33, 63, 98, 100, 165
Bladder Infection, 76
Blood Pressure, 21, 72, 74
Blue Vervain, 68
Blue Violet, 93
Boils, 135, 165
Bones, 37
Borage, 68
Bowel, 22, 24, 29, 37, 38, 40, 60, 66, 76, 82, 93, 113, 128, 137, 148, 163, 166
Brain-Damage, 16
Burns, 16
Burnshaw, Peggy 108

C

Calcium, 21
Cancer, 12, 13, 25, 31, 63, 76, 93, 135, 137, 155, 161, 162, 174
Canker, 137, 144, 183
Capsicum, 74, 97, 100, 101, 111, 113, 145, 146
Cardiovascular, 20
Cascara Sagrada, 68
Catnip, 29, 144, 171
Cayenne, 61, 166
Cedar Berries, 30
Chaparral, 63, 175
Chickweed, 68
Children, 10, 25, 34, 71, 79, 83, 86, 88, 90, 93, 95, 98, 99, 100, 104, 105, 106, 114,

Slippery Elm, 37, 61, 145
Socrates, 180, 183
Solomon, 181, 182
Spine, 42, 80, 88, 99
Splenik, Melva, 110
St. John's Wort, 68
Stephenson, Georgia, 97
Stevenson, Robert Louis, 179
Stokes, Denice, 84
Stomach, 19, 23, 28, 30, 31, 32, 38, 42, 60, 72, 77, 79, 84, 88, 134, 137, 140, 142, 149, 160, 165
Storres, Richard, 129
Story, Shirley, 130
Stratinger, Lorna, 111
Strep Infection, 128
Stress, 22, 29, 32, 38, 42, 71, 75, 79, 98, 99, 135, 138, 139, 147, 150, 151, 153, 155
Surgery, 12, 13, 14, 21, 34, 63, 75, 79, 93, 107, 113, 114, 128, 129, 169

T
Talmud, 179
Tansy, 68
Tapeworm, 161
Texture, 20, 22, 59, 98, 187
Thompson, Elaine, 141
Thyroid, 30, 31, 41, 97, 111, 113, 139, 174
Thyroid, 30
Tongue, 84, 109, 123
Toxicity, 22
Tracy, Michael, 45, 167
Tree Of Disease, 44
Trench Mouth, 137
Trichinosis, 63

Tumors, 24, 75, 97, 101

U
Ulcers, 101, 135, 137, 165
Upwall, Bessie, 145
Uric Acid, 30, 32, 38, 60, 64

V
Valerian, 145
Veranth, Ruth, 173
Vitality, 77, 81, 84, 87, 89, 109
Vitamin C, 15, 37, 64, 65, 77, 83, 85, 98, 103, 106, 109, 123, 132, 133, 143, 144, 153, 172

W
Walters, Doyle, 76, 79
Weakness, 20, 22, 23, 38, 39, 40, 43, 59, 64, 66, 101, 117, 123, 183
Webster, Daniel, 183
Wheeler, Rich, 148
Whitear, Vera, 137
Whitman, Walt, 191
Widtsoe, Leah, 14, 123
Wisdom Teeth, 85
Wood, Gloria, 137
Word of Wisdom, 86, 94, 100, 122, 123, 148
Worms, 24, 85, 155

Y
Yancey, Shirley, 106
Yellowdock, 68
Young, Brigham, 14, 178
Young, Edward, 178
Z
Ziros, Mabel U., 75

RIGHT IRIS

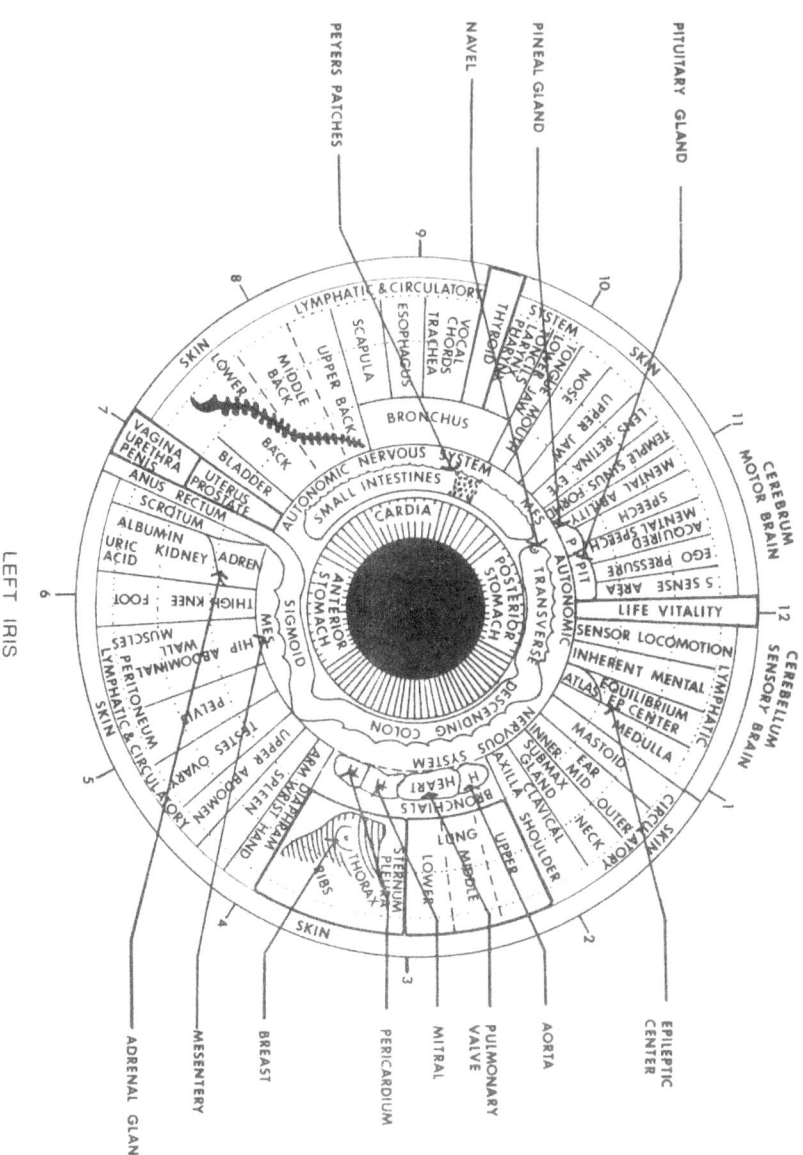

LEFT IRIS

PITUITARY GLAND

PINEAL GLAND

NAVEL

PEYERS PATCHES

CEREBRUM MOTOR BRAIN

CEREBELLUM SENSORY BRAIN

EPILEPTIC CENTER

AORTA

PULMONARY VALVE

MITRAL

PERICARDIUM

SKIN

BREAST

MESENTERY

ADRENAL GLAND

LYMPHATIC & CIRCULATORY

VOCAL CHORDS
TRACHEA
THYROID

ESOPHAGUS

SCAPULA

UPPER BACK

SKIN LOWER
MIDDLE
BACK

BRONCHUS

VAGINA
URETHRA
PENIS

BLADDER

UTERUS
PROSTATE

ANUS RECTUM

SCROTUM

ALBUMIN

URIC ACID

KIDNEY ADREN

AUTONOMIC NERVOUS SYSTEM

SMALL INTESTINES

CARDIA

POSTERIOR STOMACH

ANTERIOR STOMACH

TRANSVERSE

AUTONOMIC

SYSTEM STOMACH TONGUE MOUTH

TONSIL PARNIS PHARYNX

NOSE

UPPER JAW

LENS RETINAL EYE

TEMPLE SINUS FOREHEAD

MENTAL ABILITY

SPEECH

ACQUIRED MENTAL SPEECH

PIT

EGO PRESSURE

S SENSE AREA

LIFE VITALITY

SENSOR LOCOMOTION

INHERENT MENTAL

EQUILIBRIUM CENTER

ATLAS EP CENTER

MEDULLA

MASTOID

INNER EAR MID

SUBMAX GLAND

CLAVICAL

NECK

MAXILLA

OUTER

SHOULDER

UPPER

MIDDLE

LOWER

LUNG

BRONCHIALS

HEART

STERNUM PLEURA

THORAX

RIBS

SKIN

UPPER ABDOMEN

ARM WRIST HAND

SPLEEN

TESTES OVARY

PELVIS

LYMPHATIC & CIRCULATORY SKIN

PERITONEUM

HIP ABDOMINAL WALL

MUSCLES

THIGH KNEE FOOT

MES

SIGMOID

DESCENDING COLON

NERVOUS SYSTEM

SKIN

CIRCULATORY

LYMPHATIC

204

www.ingramcontent.com/pod-product-compliance
Lightning Source LLC
Chambersburg PA
CBHW070409290526
45791CB00005B/1689